Praise for *This Day W...*

"My wife passed away from cancer ... I think both she and I would have .... we had been able to read *This Day Won't Come Again*. I hope the book will help others facing cancer to find meaning in their lives."

—JAMES OLSON, PhD, professor of psychology
at Western University Ontario

"Scattering her gems of insight with generous abandon, these are lessons for all of us, for regardless of whether or not we have personal experience with illness, it is something that touches us all. . . . Guiding her listeners through tough spiritual terrain, Jocelyn encourages us to embrace the journey, always secure in the knowledge that we are not alone."

—MARIA L. CASE, composer and
artistic director of The Annex Singers

"This book is a revelation and a remarkable offering, not only for those facing cancer, but for anyone grappling with life's challenges. With startling honesty, humor, and a lovely compassion for the human experience, Jocelyn offers rare insight into illness and healing, and encourages a new way of seeing for readers on their own brave journeys."

—CHRISTEN SHEPHERD, death doula,
and co-author of *The Promise:
Truth from the Trenches of Adoption, Stories That Matter*

"Through the discords of cancer, Jocelyn invites us to listen for the bright, tender, and vibrant notes that carry humanity through our joy and woe. With breathtaking insight, Jocelyn's personal story, her song of life, inspires."

—JEFFREY CRITTENDEN, PhD, founding director
of the Centre for Practical Theology
and author of Leisure Resurrected

THIS
DAY
WON'T
COME
AGAIN

THIS DAY WON'T COME AGAIN

Radical Presence and Life-Threatening Illness

JOCELYN RASMUSSEN

SHE WRITES PRESS

Copyright © 2025 Jocelyn Rasmussen

All rights reserved. No part of this publication may be reproduced, distributed, or transmitted in any form or by any means, including photocopying, recording, digital scanning, or other electronic or mechanical methods, without the prior written permission of the publisher, except in the case of brief quotations embodied in critical reviews and certain other noncommercial uses permitted by copyright law. For permission requests, please address She Writes Press.

Published 2025

Printed in the United States of America

Print ISBN: 978-1-64742-938-6
E-ISBN: 978-1-64742-939-3
Library of Congress Control Number: 2025906237

For information, address:
She Writes Press
1569 Solano Ave #546
Berkeley, CA 94707

Interior design and typeset by Katherine Lloyd, The DESK
She Writes Press is a division of SparkPoint Studio, LLC.

Company and/or product names that are trade names, logos, trademarks, and/or registered trademarks of third parties are the property of their respective owners and are used in this book for purposes of identification and information only under the Fair Use Doctrine.

NO AI TRAINING: Without in any way limiting the author's [and publisher's] exclusive rights under copyright, any use of this publication to "train" generative artificial intelligence (AI) technologies to generate text is expressly prohibited. The author reserves all rights to license uses of this work for generative AI training and development of machine learning language models.

Names and identifying characteristics have been changed to protect the privacy of certain individuals.

To the scientists and researchers
the medical professionals
and caregivers all

now the ears of my ears awake and

now the eyes of my eyes are opened

—E. E. Cummings

CONTENTS

Foreword *by Dr. Akira Sugimoto* xi

Preface 1

Healing 6

The Collapse of Time 17

Cardinal Matters 30

Hope 44

Abide with Me 56

Generative Conversation 69

Work 83

Going for the Gold 94

Celebration 104

Dreaming 115

The Lover 127

Gravity 137

The Poetry of Cancer 145

Sources 149

Acknowledgments 151

About the Author 153

FOREWORD

Neuropsychologists theorize that the human brain consists of two opposing and complementary systems. The first is responsible for thinking and deals with cognitions, matters of intellect, and ideas. It is logical. The second is responsible for feeling and deals with emotions and intuition. In medical school, we are trained primarily to develop the first system, to become intellects and diagnosticians and to become experts in formulating a treatment plan. I've often referred to this as the "find the problem and fix the problem" model of medicine.

In the care of cancer patients, billions of dollars and decades of research have led to novel cancer therapies that are now allowing cancer patients to live longer and with better quality of life than ever before. However, despite these many advancements, cancer remains a life-threatening disease, and many patients will still succumb to their illness.

There are intensely frightening questions that come from living with cancer: How long will I live? What will my quality of life be? What can I expect? What can my family expect? Despite the many medical advances, a physician can still not accurately see into the future and therefore cannot answer these questions. Life for patients living with cancer means not having answers to any of these important and fundamental questions.

THIS DAY WON'T COME AGAIN

As physicians, those highly trained intellectual parts of our brains now become useless in helping patients with this kind of suffering. Therefore we are forced to depart from being fixers, authoritarians, or even relievers of suffering. We must move into being compassionate listeners, being patient and humble enough to share a space of emotional suffering with another person where we cannot diminish that suffering. I've often said to my students that the toughest cases they will encounter are not those that require a long operation or weeks of diagnostic challenges but rather those cases where nothing at all can be done to fix or alleviate the illness, where instead they will find themselves sharing space and time with a patient whose suffering cannot be diminished.

The many years of medical training do not prepare doctors for this task. Instead, the greatest teachers of this work are actually our patients. Not our professors, not our textbooks, but our patients.

I have had the privilege of caring for Jocelyn as her oncologist for several years. In her characteristically humble way she will say that her journey has in many ways been no different than anyone else's. What is remarkable however is how extremely hard she has worked to find meaning in all that she has experienced. To lean into the suffering. To feel it as completely as possible, to explore it and to learn from it.

This book, written by an individual suffering from cancer, is Jocelyn's own personal, soulful, reflective, and loving account of the thoughts and feelings that she has experienced throughout her journey. I hope the grace, courage, struggle, pain, joy, clarity, and peace that she has found while en route shine a light that will guide others to find the path to their own inner peace.

FOREWORD

Dr. Akira Sugimoto, *gynecologic oncologist at London Health Sciences Centre and the London Regional Cancer Program, is the director of the Fellowship Training Program in Gynecologic Oncology in the Department of Obstetrics and Gynecology at the University of Western Ontario. He leads the design of a comprehensive care pathway for ovarian cancer patients and participates in the Communities of Practice Initiative with Cancer Care Ontario.*

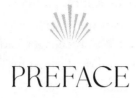

PREFACE

I was raised on a family farm under an endless Saskatchewan sky. My favorite perch was on a hill covered in ancient stone carvings of animal tracks, turtles, human hands, feet, and heads, and at least one complete human being. Sitting there you could look farther than you could see and imagine the world had no edges, only horizons. The night sky had as many stars as the prairie had blades of grass. Everything was countless. It made me a dreamer.

I loved to watch dancing loops of light all around me. They were beautiful and entrancing. I noticed one went into my forehead and my mind began wrapping words around it. It seemed to me these loops were thoughts, and some of them became mine. One way to describe my time with cancer is to say I have reentered the realm of dancing light and radiant thoughts. It is like being at the core of a sphere and being able to travel any radius to a point on its surface, like finding life can move in any direction—beside, behind, in front, above, or below—in the blink of an eye. This is both liberating and disorienting. It is nothing I would ever have wished for and not something I now would wish away.

Childhood was harder for me than cancer has been. Our family home was not a house of hate, but neither was it a made-for-television ideal. We were eight strong-willed people, each with our own versions of the stories that happened beneath one small roof. I had painful eczema, was susceptible to sickness, and by the time I was a teenager had developed allergies to just about everything on the farm. This meant I could not be outside with the others feeding cattle or working in the fields, but there was plenty of work to go around, and all six children learned to do our share. My chores mostly involved housework and cooking. One day while I was helping Mama make her bed we were chatting away and she said she and Papa had wanted only four children. She saw my little face drop and my eyes fill with tears—I was child number five. She quickly said they were so happy that I had been born.

Years later, as I was trying to understand the roots of a lifelong depression and suicidal ideation, I learned that a mother's emotions during pregnancy have an effect on the unborn child. I remembered what my mother had told me and thought of how difficult it must have been for my parents to be expecting another child when there already was not enough to go around. I was grateful she had let it slip. It helped me to forgive myself and to have more compassion for all of us. By that time I had experienced more than enough of my mother's love to know I truly was wanted.

Doing household chores was perfect for me. I worked as hard and fast as I could in order to steal a little time to play the piano and sing. From the age of three when that magnificent, upright grand piano arrived, it was my solace and portal to dreaming. Everything else disappeared as my little fingers learned the magical order of keys that created the music already in my ears and voice. I did not formally study music during my school-age years, so I was unqualified to pursue a classical music degree at university. Eventually I found my way to a jazz school where I studied vocal performance and composition. I later

PREFACE

studied classical singing at colleges in the United States, but after years of dealing with thyroid disease and chronic allergies, the hourglass was running out of sand. I reluctantly surrendered my dreams of a performing career to become a singing teacher. I was both surprised and grateful to learn I do not have to be the one singing in order to be happy. I love teaching with all my heart and soul, and I continue composing and performing on the side. My passion for the human voice has never diminished and continues to lead me through life.

For years I lived in New York City and eventually applied for permanent residence. When my petition was denied, my O-1 visa also was terminated. I moved back to Canada and lost everything except who I had become. I found myself in my mid-fifties with no husband or children, no home, no work, and no pension. It occurred to me I also had no overhead, no dependents, no obligations, and no debt. I was in the perfect position to do something new. I could use that freedom any way I chose.

I decided life was giving me a sabbatical and poured myself into writing my first book. My father died. I met a choreographer and casting director with whom I started an integrated arts program for children. I was diagnosed with cancer. We closed the business and I began teaching privately again. My mother died. By the time I began cancer treatment I was up to my hips in illness and loss. Fortunately, events that caused me to return to Canada gave me access to universal health care with no deductible, co-pay, or conditions. I now needed that more than other material assets that had gone by the wayside.

My life has had times of difficulty when I could not see the light, but in hindsight it has always seemed to be magical and blessed. I might have felt sad and isolated during childhood, but I had that piano and the sky and dreaming to see me through. In later years I felt more than a little disappointed that I never married and had children, but living independently, without the demands of a family, I have been able to explore wherever my curiosity and passion led. While most people I know grow through building a marriage and raising children, I have developed through endless effort to stay afloat while enduring solitude and rigorous hours of reflection. It is tempting to look at someone else's path and think it is better, but that is like saying the heart works harder than the lungs. Each life is like a cell in the collective body of humanity, and it is enough for each of us to live into our own design.

The way each of us navigates cancer is a chapter in the healing story of humanity. Many new thoughts arise because of it, and the experience can change how we have always thought about things, including memories. Those of us living with cancer find we are constantly learning, but not necessarily the same things as one another. We are alike in surprising ways and different in countless others. Every person has a story to tell about having cancer, and although they are all different and unique, they are the way we come together to create a circle of knowledge.

On the following pages is my story. I began sharing it as a series of talks I gave about hope and healing at Glebe Road United Church in Toronto. I wrote the talks not only for people with cancer but also for anyone else with a life-threatening or chronic illness. They are for caregivers and loved ones who are as profoundly affected as those with illness. We all are engaged with the demands of illness and healing, though we do not always feel we are in it together. We may not always relate to one another's experiences, but we can still be inspired by each other's insights. I could not have guessed how much these talks would support my own healing, and I have been humbled by the degree to which they have supported others.

As an artist, I mine the raw experience of my life to interpret and express what has beauty and power for me. This practice

PREFACE

colors the way I see what happens to me and predisposes me to a certain kind of reflection. I realize cancer is not a doorway to creativity for everyone. When you do not have health care or other resources needed to survive, cancer is a frightening disruption and a recipe for becoming overwhelmed. It is precisely because I have had a different and radiant experience that others have encouraged me to write about it. I am not trying to give advice or present steps to take for healing. I offer this text as one offers any art. It is meant to be company and to encourage others to cherish their own experience. It is my love song to life and to you.

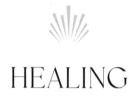

HEALING

Tuesday, May 28, 2013. I looked out the window to see what kind of day it was promising to be. I heard myself say in a matter-of-fact voice, "Oh. I have cancer." It was a startling moment and I had no idea where the thought came from. I could not remember my dreams and had not had a single symptom that would make me imagine I had any kind of illness. I fell into a spacious stillness, a timeless quiet. It occurred to me there might be something better about my dying sooner rather than later. Perhaps something significant would occur or be avoided. Not that cancer means you will die, but it *is* the second leading cause of death globally, so it is not surprising many of us immediately consider that option.

I need a miracle, I thought. *If it could be a spontaneous remission, that would be amazing. If it needs to be a cure through medical treatment, I can do that.* Then I surprised myself by thinking, *If it's a shift out of this life and into whatever's next, that'll be okay too.* Once that sank in, I had one final thought: *If I'm allowed to ask for anything, I'd like the most love and grace that could possibly come through my life to be spent before I die, whenever that is.*

The medical diagnosis came a couple months after my curious awakening on that cloudy May morning. Ovarian cancer had arrived as my next path of learning, as a new discipline for discovery and growth. I did not seem to be having a spontaneous remission, so I embraced medical treatment. There was no guarantee of a cure, but it would at least give me time.

Nothing about cancer has felt like a mistake. I know there are larger forces at work than my hopes and dreams, and there is no reason why I should not be one of the 30 percent of women who will have some form of cancer in their lives. Each and every wonderful person on my care team seems to be someone I was destined to meet. It is as though we have pieces of each other we have been saving for just this moment. I have an exceedingly wise, compassionate healer I call my doctor and an angel I call my social worker. At a clinic that sometimes feels to me more like a temple than a hospital, I receive the most up-to-date care available. Every nurse, technician, administrative assistant, janitor, and volunteer supports my healing in both traditional and surprising ways. We have had the most wonderful conversations about family, marriage, children, work, the world, hopes and dreams . . . and cancer. When fellow patients share their terrible and tender stories, they become my heroes and inspiration. Family, friends, and students also have revealed themselves as miracle workers in the process of my treatment.

I consider everyone I have encountered because of cancer to be a guide of sorts. Each has ferried me across a river of circumstance to a new territory within myself and exposed me to the world around me in ways I never thought about before I met them. Together we have become storytellers, partners in a mystery school where we inscribe our days with sometimes visionary and often desperate prayers. They are unsuspecting participants in the miracle I asked for that gray May morning.

Along with everything the world of Western medicine offers to treat cancer, there is a universe of complementary remedies, diets, mindsets and meditations, rituals and shamans. I love that everyone can choose the form of treatment that feels best to them, and with an epidemic like cancer it is most assuredly time to pull out all the stops. I might have misunderstood, but it seemed to me some complementary or spiritual approaches were asking me to come to terms with how I have failed to live up to my potential, or how life has damaged me, or where deficiencies in my attitude and self-care may have caused my disease. My brother, the joker, pointed out I am the one in the family who tries so hard to be healthy, but I am the one with cancer. It is true. I have long been into wellness and alternative approaches. I quit my addictions, I exercise and take nutritional supplements, I seek support to remain mentally and emotionally balanced, and I actually answer the questions in the self-help books I read. No one could accuse me of not at least trying to overcome my problematic defects of character. All the actions I took did not prevent my getting cancer, so I changed my approach and embraced medical treatment. Later on I would learn I am genetically predisposed to ovarian cancer, and something turned that gene on. The gene is quite prevalent in my family, and it gets turned on rather a lot. I used to say cancer was my family's disease of choice. In spite of that I never imagined I might succumb to it. In the words of Mark Twain, "Denial ain't just a river in Egypt."

As I began sorting through what to do to treat my illness, looking at both Western medicine and all the healthful living in which I had engaged, I wondered if there might be a difference between being healed and being cured. Although the two terms are used interchangeably, I think of curing as being the end of disease, and being healed as feeling at peace with the process of one's life. Healing can happen at any stage of an illness and is not dependent on being cured. It is a state of acceptance, a sense of wholeness that includes joy and sadness, success and failure, health and sickness. My loves and heroes dying from cancer were no less wise, compassionate, or at peace because they were riddled with disease; in fact, it was often quite the opposite. They were the most glorious people I know in the way they embraced death, which is the final and great healing of every life. Cancer does not necessarily care if we exercise and drink green smoothies. It does not care if we meditate and do community service. These things and countless others have at least anecdotally led to a cure for some people, but not for everyone who does them. The same is true of surgery, chemotherapy, radiation, and immunotherapy. Sometimes these treatments effect a cure and sometimes not. After years of research, too many people defy every finding to claim that any approach, whether traditional or alternative medicine, could be certain for everyone. Cancer is different every time, and whatever approach we choose requires great faith.

The very definition of faith means I have no idea what the outcome will be. Faith is not something I practice in order to get a desired outcome. I practice it knowing that every outcome is, eventually, going to deliver something that can be used for good. In the great mystery teachings, we are encouraged to practice prayer and meditation in order to rise to a metaphorical mountaintop where we may gain illuminated perspective and inspiration, where we are invited to release our burdens and longings and receive a sense of unconditional love in return. When one engages in a spiritual tradition, there is often a requirement to practice certain disciplines designed to strengthen character and cultivate one's inner life. People who engage in these practices are referred to as disciples on a path of learning. A discipleship with healing reconciles the mystical experience of infinite love and perfection with the very human experience of faith, whether our illness is cured or not.

Healing is rooted in a reverence for what is. It flows from gratitude for five delicious and very earthly senses that also are capable of pain and suffering. Healing turns each corner with a kaleidoscope imagination that adores a good adventure and is no stranger to trouble. Healing flows from a heart that can be true to itself no matter the storm that is breaking. Healing rises on the wings of stories that have been a lifetime in the making, that are sweetened by the memories of cherished and dangerous loves. Healing tenderly weaves the dazzling and frayed threads of our hopes and dreams into the astonishing tapestry of our days.

Healing is not any one thing we do. It is a transformative gift that unfolds as we open into it. As with illness, the constellation of healing is never twice the same. The creative force of life fashions it anew for each of us with indestructible love and unstoppable grace. When we come together for healing, we find in one another the eyes, hands, and heart of the sacred in human expression.

Being healed means we will experience our fullness and our place in creation no matter the circumstance. It means we may *receive* our breath with gratitude instead of *taking* it with frenzy, and we can spend our life generously for the purpose that is ours alone to fulfill. I have lived a very busy life trying to make my dreams come true and have complained more than enough that not a one of them ever did. A few years ago I realized I have a life better than my unfulfilled dreams because I did not know enough to dream the life I have. I was playing piano and singing with a group of elders who have Alzheimer's disease. We had just started singing when, to my surprise, children came in from a neighboring day school to dance with the elders. Tears were streaming down my face because I could not believe I was part of something so tender and joyful. It was powerful for me in a way no staged performance ever was. I had been trying fiercely to create the career of my dreams. Meanwhile, life had been turning me into someone willing to serve the power of music, wherever it takes me.

HEALING

One day while pondering how I could describe the mystery of living with disease and the grace of healing I was experiencing, I began to see many different images of water. At first it was running in a quiet river. I saw it being imbibed by animals and osmosed by plants. Then there were rapids and a waterfall along its journey to the ocean. It evaporated and traveled as clouds to distant lands. It was frozen for thousands of years on polar ice caps and trapped for millennia inside giant crystals. It was hydrating algae in stagnant ponds and cooling nuclear waste. And it was all precious, life-giving water.

Who would say to the water in the rapids, "Dashing against those rocks is irresponsible—you could get bounced to shore and end up in the belly of a bear"? Or suggest to water in the ocean, "You've lost your identity and need to learn how to stand on your own two feet"? Or call water in polar ice caps rigid and tell it to get a life, or accuse clouds of being flighty and insist they figure out how to get grounded? Who would explain to water in stinking ponds or used to cool industrial waste that it has bad karma from a past life or failed to forgive a difficult childhood? And when water floods the plains, who would declare, "That water needs to get control of itself and establish some boundaries"?

This is not a perfect analogy. A human being is infinitely more complex than a droplet of water. And our very human choices definitely have cause and effect. The point is the law of cause and effect is bigger than any one of us and is not the entirety of what is at play. The interrelatedness of life stretches across all of existence and draws us into the mystery of creation. Whatever the source of creation might be, I have never believed we would be created with the power of choice and then be punished for exercising it. We learn through the experiences we create and also from the ones we bump into that others have created. In so many of our attempts to name the cause of illness

THIS DAY WON'T COME AGAIN

or determine where to place the blame, we simply suffer grief and heartache. Being cured or healed is not dependent on laying blame or judging the value of a life in its evolutionary moment. There are reasons great and small for where we find ourselves, and their purpose is not to make us guilty. Every circumstance is to help us become more aware, to help us make new choices with greater understanding. Life evolves through us, with or without disease, and we have value to bring to it before, during, and after we get sick.

Illness moves in with a big suitcase. It unpacks layers of struggle, pain, doubt, and hopelessness. It takes things out of the closet and does not put them back. It invades your privacy and interferes with your plans. It demands your attention and leaves you feeling exhausted. Then, just as it has turned your life upside down and inside out, it reveals itself as an inspired messenger. This same illness calls you to the guidance that resides within all of us. Together, illness and inexplicable life force unlock door after door to unexplored courage, resilience, humor, intuition, compassion, wisdom, humility, willingness, and grit. They help us to let go of fears, weaknesses, and delusions that no longer serve us. Cancer is for some people to have the same way they have talents and limitations. Our choice may not be in whether or not we have it but rather in how we live with it.

I do not feel like I am dying. I feel like I have time in me, but since I initially was given rather slim odds of being cured, I decided I should write a bucket list. I sat with pen and paper for a while and finally realized I had nothing to put on it. I trust the process of my life, and I assume that if I need to finish certain things, I will be here until they are accomplished. There is much I can imagine doing if my health allows, but the old self-importance has been drained out of me. Nothing about what I can do seems essential. It is simply possible. This

HEALING

day is an invitation, not an imperative. It is not that I have no regrets or have not messed up as much as I have achieved. I did so many stupid things it is a miracle I lived long enough to get cancer. I have not always done the good I could, and I almost cannot bear the harm I have generated. It has been humbling and humiliating to have so much to learn and to be so slow on the uptake at times.

I also have done some good, and I bless the wonderful people in my life who have made a point of letting me know. With the benefit of time and reflection, I have been able to see how my weaknesses and shortcomings forced me to develop my strengths and talents. Despite what I had observed in others I knew and loved who had cancer, I knew nothing about what it would ask of me. Was I willing to live it wholeheartedly without knowing how my story would end? Could I be not in the grips of cancer but rather in the throes of life? Could I go into the mystery of this day as though it has no end, no beginning, no time but this extravagant unknowable moment? Could I follow the thread of treatment I choose for what I will become as a result of it and not regret the other threads not chosen? Perhaps those other options would be neither better nor worse but only different. My relationship with cancer opened with a blank page. I felt the most expansive I have ever felt in the whole of my life. Everything seemed possible, and nothing seemed possible too.

When I returned to Canada, one of the first things I did was visit my parents. Living far away meant I did not see them often, and they seemed to age ever more quickly between visits. I had an opportunity to take a writing retreat in Switzerland and they very much wanted me to go. When they took me to the plane, Papa said it might be the last time we see each other. I made it home three beautiful days before he died. I cherish those days as much as any I have ever lived. He was a Christian

THIS DAY WON'T COME AGAIN

believer, and I reminded him that the Bible says God knows us before we are born. I told him I thanked God for putting me with my perfect earthly father so I could become the woman I was born to be. He was no longer talking, but he squeezed my hand again and again. Then I reminded us both he was going to become pure light and he would be in a world of glorious radiance. It would be the most peaceful, exquisitely beautiful experience he had ever had, and all he had to do was go toward that light. Again he squeezed and squeezed my hand. That was our final goodbye. While Mama was singing the hymn "Coming Home," he left his body.

Mama had her routine, which I learned during the months I stayed with her after Papa died. Every morning she got up, put breakfast on the table, and said her morning prayers before eating. Five days before my second surgery, my niece found Mama sitting at the table, her hands folded in her lap, her breakfast uneaten. My brother called to tell me she had left her body during her morning prayers.

The news of her death did not immediately sink in. I went back to my computer in an altered state. I had just connected an external sound system and thought I should make sure everything was working. What should I play? I decided to log on to YouTube. Once there I thought, *Why not some yodeling?* Up came a song called "Yodeling in Heaven." Under any other circumstance I cannot imagine I would have chosen this. It felt as though some other force had guided me to the song, perhaps the spirit of my mother's love, perhaps an intuition of what I needed in that moment. You see, Mama used to yodel for us when we were children. As I listened to the singer's touching story about her mother's death and their bond to yodeling, I moved out of the fog of shock into my own trembling heart. It broke as the news of Mama's death became real to me.

HEALING

It was three days before Canadian Thanksgiving. My surgery was scheduled to take place immediately after Thanksgiving, and it seemed impossible to bury Mama in time for me to fly to Saskatchewan and back before the operation. I told my family to do whatever they had to and that I would join the funeral virtually. While they were busy making arrangements, I felt as though Mama was dictating her eulogy to me. I typed it up and emailed it to them, writing, "Use as much or as little of this as you choose. I'm not sure what you have in mind, but thought it might help." The return email said, "It's perfect and you'll be giving it." My family had found a way to have the funeral service on Thanksgiving Day so I could be there. Mama had told me years earlier about a song she wanted sung at her funeral. I had bought the music but never learned it. Thankfully I had time before my flight.

The morning after the funeral, at an hour even too early for roosters and babies, I boarded the plane for the return flight. The following day I had a radical hysterectomy. I was grateful my parents would not have to live through this illness with me, but I have never wanted them more. Even though I had felt misunderstood and unacceptable to my parents for much of my life, we had managed to resolve our differences and express our love in later years. I learned very quickly just how much I had been relying on them for my sense of security and unconditional love in the world. Not only had I lost my work and life in New York City; I now had lost my parents and my health. Part of my healing was going to involve standing on my own two feet as never before.

I find it interesting that my cancer actually was not on or in my ovaries at all but in my left fallopian tube. It behaves exactly like ovarian cancer and has the same treatment, but it is rarer. All my life I had worked tirelessly to realize my dreams, to birth my projects, but everything had failed to find its support in the external world. It was as though my life itself had a blocked fallopian tube. Some might look at that blocked tube and say I created the cancer with all my failures. This is something alternative teachings had me wondering about. However, my first surgeon said the tube could have been blocked my entire life without my knowing it. I vaguely remember a doctor mentioning it, maybe in my twenties. I never tried to have children, so I gave it no more thought. Since cancer has come, that blockage has been removed, I have published two books, a new album of songs I have composed is in the world and earning money for ovarian cancer research, and I teach singing as a transformational practice rather than merely as an art form. Perhaps undergoing cancer treatment has helped me to birth some of my creativity. Regardless of how I look at it, cancer for me is not something to resent. Perhaps I needed a lifetime of preparation to do this work and I am going to be able to manifest more quickly now. There is no proof it would have been better to write and record projects sooner, nor is it clear I had the wisdom and experience at an earlier time in my life to do it as well as I might now. There is no assurance I would be more productive as I age if I had manifested more in my youth. All we can know for certain is that my life would be different.

Perhaps the greatest and most powerful aspect of healing is the new ways we learn to look at things. Each and every one of us will have a unique point of view on disease, and we all will interpret matters according to our own moment and place in evolution. That interpretation will work on us and with us. As we learn to express it through the way we speak and live, it will become part of our legacy. Whether we view our experience with cancer as tragedy, destiny, or opportunity, it will be our contribution to humanity's collective healing story. No matter what, when all is said and done, our life will have meaning and beauty.

THE COLLAPSE
OF TIME

A few landed softly on outstretched branches, others skirted trees to rest on gardens below, some hit sidewalks to be trampled by after-school chaos, and a multitude wreaked havoc in the streets. On the sofa, recovering from a round of chemotherapy, I stared out the window and slipped into a state of accidental concentration. I became aware of a subtle, energetic grid within which every tiny flake of a massive snowstorm had its own path and lifespan. Each was utterly unique not only in its structure but also in its destiny. One was heading true as a plumb line toward the driveway when a tiny current swept it horizontally and delivered it to a papery sprig. Another graced a bird's crest until a flutter of plumage launched it anew. Down the street some flakes were not even falling. Sucked into a vortex between buildings, the spiraling updraft carried them concentrically higher until, above the rooftops, the pattern of the vortex dissipated and they spun off to meander again toward earth. Within this cosmic blueprint, nothing about a single one of those little flakes falling outside my window seemed careless or mistaken. I watched for hours.

When I returned my gaze to inside the room, I saw the grid everywhere. Every object in the room was placed within it and vibrated with energy. Later, when a friend came to visit, I saw that she too moved and vibrated within this energetic grid. As she spoke, she began to appear to me as different people from different periods in history. They were different sexes, ages, and ethnicities. After a while, she turned into pure light. There was no human form, only radiance. Science has revealed that everyone is a constellation of generations with the map of their lineage in their DNA. Now it seems to me everyone also exists as radiant energy that is beyond these physical forms.

According to Native American cultures, everything we do affects the seven generations before us and the seven to come after us. Cause and effect play out not only within the span of an individual life but over generations. When we look at things this way, we understand that we are working on matters set in motion by our ancestors and their legacy is in our hands. Something that looks like their failure may create the need for a brilliant innovation in our generation, which ends up moving humanity in a positive direction. At the same time we are putting new elements into play with which our offspring will have to contend. When I lost track of time and perceptual prejudice, I was able to see an expanse of generations influencing a single life.

When I first realized I had cancer and was considering the value of a long life compared to one cut short, I thought of Terry Fox. He was eighteen years old when cancer came and took his leg from above the knee. Of all the possible choices available to him, including despair, he settled on the "Marathon of Hope." Imagine the sensation of each breath as he ran the equivalent of a full marathon every day, all while enduring the pain of a prosthetic limb. Before he could finish his cross-Canada run, cancer came back and took Terry's life, but decades later the "Marathon of Hope" continues. It has raised more than $850 million since 1980, and there is no end in sight. Because of the choices he made, Terry Fox's life was as miraculous to me as it would have been if he had had a spontaneous remission. If I had met him, would I have seen his radiant body, the essential part of his being that took those inspiring actions to help so many others for generations to come, despite his personal suffering? Every week I see people at the clinic who are living from the radiant aspect of their being. They are the kind of people we describe as bright lights. They are not waiting to be cured. They use their creative spirit to bring love and goodness to the moments they have right now. We will never know how much more Terry might have achieved if he had lived longer, but through the run his creative spirit is still very much present in our lives, and one way or another everyone's creative spirit lives on. Our legacy also can be an expression of healing carried from generation to generation in the hands of others. That is why many patients enter clinical trials. They know the experiments are randomized and that they might receive a placebo, but they hope that even if they themselves are not helped, in the future others will be because they chose to participate.

Time seems to stand still when we are deeply engaged in a creative work or entranced as I was with the snow. It seems to stop altogether when we are falling, or in a serious accident, or receive life-altering news of any kind, but these scenarios have absolutely no effect on real time. Five seconds is five seconds. However, faced with a dire circumstance, the mind shifts into an altered state in which it is able to perceive everything that is possible in an instant rather than the one thing it would normally focus on in a linear fashion from moment to moment. Suddenly, in a state of complete and radical presence, a moment is an eternity, and every option within it becomes available. Eternity is not endless time but the end of time. Once we are removed from linear time and fall into an altered state, one of the alternative dimensions we can perceive is that an illness never happened. When we begin again to perceive time, we

THIS DAY WON'T COME AGAIN

might learn we have been fully restored to a state of health. It is as though we enter the sphere I described in the preface. We travel to the center along the path of one radius, and then we exit by a different radius to a healthy point in our lives. This is one way to envision what we call a spontaneous remission or a miracle.

Where we tend to err is in defining miracles according to whether or not we get what we want, whether our desire would be a spontaneous cure, financial abundance, a soulmate, or a mystical experience. In evolutionary creation everything is possible, including natural disaster and all manner of calamity. We measure our faith in the miraculous not only by what we intentionally manifest but also by our capacity to see the possibility in what arises when our plans are blown to smithereens.

I had lived my life consumed by time and unaware of the possibilities that could be available if its structure collapsed into a radiant experience of presence. I always needed more time and I could never figure out where it had gone. Seconds gathered into days. Page after calendar page, months ran to seasons and years. I drove around in the latest model of a game plan and ignored the present while I was waiting for the light to change. When cancer came for me, time lost its power. It does not matter if the end of my life is decades away or tomorrow. I am on another plan now. This moment I am privileged to share with you as you read my words is defined by our shared awareness in it, not by a date on a calendar. It holds within it all that has led up to it and all that will come from it. It is complete. There is nowhere else to be and nothing else to do. However, being present does not mean we never reflect on the past or plan for the future. This is another aspect of presence that influences the process of healing.

If I am remembering the past, I am bringing it into the present. If I am planning for the future, I am bringing it into

THE COLLAPSE OF TIME

the present. The question is, am I completely focused on it, or is it a distracting background noise to something else I had intended to focus on? For example, am I somewhat engaged in conversation but unable to deeply listen because I am embarrassed about what I said fifteen minutes ago? Am I planning lunch while doing yoga or thinking about how to get to the train on time while I am in a meeting? In these cases I am not present because presence is not a location on a timeline—it is an undivided state of being. It is important to be able to bring the past into the present, to reflect on it, learn from it, and heal from it. It can be important to bring the future into the present and to plan for it with loving intention. It can also be crucial to abandon what we think we know based on the past and to surrender our intentions for what we think we need to do. Awareness divided between multiple time zones leaves one scattered and unable to attend to what is taking place now. It is the opposite of what happens when falling or faced with a crisis. An aspect of healing is the experience of feeling one's whole self in one place at one time.

Another way I experience a collapse of time and a characteristic of healing is when seemingly random, unrelated events that occur over an extended period of time suddenly connect in a moment and create a sense of meaning. A few years ago, at high noon on the hottest day of the summer in New York City, I suddenly felt compelled to stop my work and go Rollerblading. I overruled that ridiculous impulse. I was not going to Rollerblade during the hottest hour on the hottest day of the year. But the agitation simply would not dissipate. In a huff I decided if I was going to have to do it, I was going to have a slice of pizza first. Pizza? I almost never ate pizza, and certainly not in hot weather. That would normally be a salad day. Outside the deli a young man was panhandling. I offered to buy him a slice and asked him to choose his toppings. He said just cheese would be okay. I asked him if he was sure, said he could have anything he wanted. He added a couple toppings. I had him choose a beverage as well. When I went to pay, the young man serving us said he would pay for the homeless man's drink out of his tip jar. I knew he was not earning the king's ransom, and I was deeply moved by his gesture. I thanked him.

I thought that must be it and decided I could go back home. However, I still had that agitation to go Rollerblading. I have learned to heed this kind of feeling as a form of guidance, so I headed to the park. In a city of eight million people there was almost no one else on the path, and certainly no one else Rollerblading. About a half mile along, the asphalt was covered with sand the wind had blown from the baseball diamond. A year before I had come up behind a group of people in this very location. Because of them I had not seen the sand and did a face-plant that knocked the wind out of me. This time I stopped and carefully stepped my way over it. As I was doing so, a park ranger came up to me and asked if I was okay. I explained the issue with the sand, and she said they would get it cleaned up right away. In the remaining years I lived near that park, I never saw sand on that path again.

As I skated back home, I remembered how upset I had been the previous year after I had fallen. I had wondered what I was supposed to learn from that. I could not see how it fit into the larger scheme of things until a full year later. Before this scorching summer day I had never seen a ranger in that park, and I never saw one again. Until I met the ranger, Rollerblading at high noon on the hottest day of the year made no sense. Now it seemed as though everything had conspired to get a message to her, including having pizza and buying a slice for a homeless man. Without that scenario I would have arrived too early for the encounter with the ranger. Even more interesting to me was that without my fall the year before, I would have had

THE COLLAPSE OF TIME

no message to give her. I have often wondered how that story continued. Was a potentially traumatic skating fall prevented? Was anything of value achieved as a result of events unfolding the way they did for me? Apparently, it is not something I need to know.

Things may happen today that seem confusing or upsetting, but they might turn into something positive and beautiful with hindsight. If, in a near or distant future, an experience is going to seem like part of the grace of my life, I assume it is part of the grace of my life today. I do not experience cancer as a problem or a mistake. It is simply a quality of my life at present. Because of it I have met an entire community of heroes and healers. Every interaction with them seems like a divine setup, a moment that is occurring just for us. It is another way time collapses and healing takes place.

The thing that never goes away in any moment is the opportunity to choose. We are created for our choices, and they matter. It is just that they are not the only things that matter. The laws of the universe and the process of human development within those laws are perpetual. There are elements of time of which we are consciously aware—our own past and future concerns. There are also influences in our personality that are unconscious—our genetic inheritance and the teachings we absorb from our environment during the early, preconscious years of our lives when we are socialized to live by the values passed from generation to generation. There are influences on us from our social and cultural collectives—our unconscious connections to one another. All of these elements affect our choices.

When we heed the prompting of an agitating spirit, we are lifted out of the linear progressions of reflection and planning and are more able to follow inexplicable or uncomfortable impulses without knowing where they are taking us or why.

THIS DAY WON'T COME AGAIN

We might be the friend or the perfect stranger who makes a difference in someone's life as events connect us to one another in ways that at first blush seem as accidental as falling snow. We all have had the experience of someone being on our mind and thinking we should give them a call. When we do, we learn that something pivotal is happening in their lives and we are able to support their experience. When we do not, we find out later and wish we had acted on our intuition.

I was invited to two holiday parties on the same day. One host lived in an exclusive neighborhood and said I would meet influential people who might be able to help my career. The other was hosting a potluck for recovering addicts and wanted to provide some hope and cheer for them. I made a fruit salad and went to the potluck.

I surveyed the crowd. They looked pretty dismal. I sank into an empty spot on a bench. A six-year-old girl had her mother's cell phone and took an extreme close-up of my nose. We laughed at how peculiar it looked. She was wearing a little pink T-shirt that said, "Daddy's Girl."

"Are you Daddy's girl?"

"Daddy's dead."

"Oh. When did he die?"

"Six months ago."

"Do you miss him?"

"I keep his picture by my bed and pray for him every night."

"Do you know he hears your prayers, and he loves you very much?"

She sat down beside me and pulled my arm around her waist, and we stayed like that for the rest of the party. On my bike ride home, I was flooded with gratitude that I had chosen what I might be able to *give* to that day over what I might be able to *get* from it. I could not imagine a more abundant experience than the one I had just had. In that moment it was as

THE COLLAPSE OF TIME

though a huge thunderclap went off in my head. It was followed by a crystal-clear message: if I had gone to the other party with the spirit of giving instead of from a place of need, I would have had a meaningful experience there as well.

We often call death accidental, as it had been for this little girl's father, or unexplained as it is with many others. How long we live seems to be out of our hands, but whether we live in faith or fear, whether we live for what we can give or for what we can get, is a moment-to-moment choice. Our choices may not cure us, but there is healing in the intentions that govern our choosing.

A few months before she died, my friend had what was supposed to be a simple procedure to release the pressure of a tumor and allow her kidney to drain. The doctor said it would take fifteen to twenty minutes, but three hours later she still had not returned to her hospital room where I was waiting with her daughter and grandchildren. Later she told me that, when she had regained consciousness, doctors and nurses surrounded her looking worried and asked her if she was okay. She told me she had a beautiful dream during the procedure. She had gone to a glorious place where she was enveloped by indescribable bliss and had not wanted to come back. My friend was fiercely determined and did everything possible to live, but after that day she knew when the time came, she would be ready to trade the pain and procedures of cancer treatment for the ecstasy she had just experienced.

I have heard it said that at the moment of death, the spirit is liberated from the body like a genie from a lamp. Time enters eternity and form becomes light. Those of us left behind are shifted into that falling state of awareness, that all-consuming focus where, try as we might, we can think of nothing else. Our beloved has left the material world and the only way to be near them is through our radiant vision. We engage presence as never before and find possibilities within it that we have not been aware of.

A common recommendation when we are in need of healing is to slow down. Even though cancer moves very fast, once we have it, many of us are forced to move more slowly through the period of treatment and recovery. After my day with the snowfall and the shifts in perception that resulted from it, I vowed never to move too quickly again. I made a commitment to seek radical presence and radiant vision. So far, this shift has not cured my cancer, but it has made me much more susceptible to both intuition and wisdom. It has meant I am more available for a phone call or an in-person visit with a friend. It has meant I fuss less about helping my students jump through hoops or over hurdles and focus more on holding the space for them to develop their unique voices in their own time. I recognize not everyone has the luxury of slowing down, nor would I claim the authority to say it is something everyone should want or need.

Being in our radiance does not mean we control time. That is not the purpose of a life or its radiance. At our bravest and best we bring love and grace into time in a way that simultaneously supports our individual design and our collective evolution. Releasing that grace generates healing but does not mean we will be cured. Conversely, people can be cured and wait a long time to experience healing. I met a woman who had been in remission for seventeen years. She said for the first fourteen years she expected to die and did nothing but live in fear and anger. Three years ago she finally decided it looked like she was going to live and she had better get on with it. The last three years had been the most vibrant and fulfilling ever, and she was excited for her days. This is what the structure of time allows us. I hesitate to look on her fearful time as wasted years. I remember hearing if you do not stop looking for something before you find it, then all the time you spent looking is

THE COLLAPSE OF TIME

not wasted. While whatever this woman was doing all those years might have been unconscious, I have faith that something powerful was being accomplished, and that from an enlightened point of view it could look good to her as well as to us.

Sometimes the smallest stories reveal as much as pivotal events do about the way things fall together over the arc of time to create meaning and healing in our lives. One fall while I was visiting a friend in another city, the crystal fell out of an earring I was wearing, one of a pair I had received as a gift. I looked everywhere but was unable to find it on that richly patterned carpet. I put what was left of the set in a small pouch and got on with the rest of the weekend. A couple days later I was packed up and wheeling my suitcase out of the bedroom when the light caught something on the floor. There was the crystal. When I got home, I decided to transfer the earrings to a small box I would use to take them to the jeweler for repair. I dropped the fine gold hook portion of the broken earring. Down on my knees I searched for it, running my hands over the fluffy rug, under furniture, farther than it could possibly have gone. I shook the rug, but nothing fell out. It had simply vanished.

The following spring I decided to take my laptop to the balcony to get a little fresh air while working. I also made some popcorn to snack on. I soon discovered, as the pieces began blowing around the balcony, that popcorn is not the ideal outdoor food for a windy day. As I picked up the scattered puffs, right there, next to one, was the lost hook for the earring. The hook must have fallen from that fluffy rug, which I would have shaken over the railing of the balcony when I did the weekly cleaning. It is a tiny miracle that it fell out before I reached the railing, given it had stayed put when I had shaken the rug quite vigorously in the bedroom. In the world of miniature moments, I made a goofy choice to eat popcorn outside on a windy day and found my earring hook. In the world of pivotal life events,

I was denied permanent residence in another country, my entire life was uprooted, and I came home to the health care that saved my life. *A Course in Miracles* says there is no order in the size of miracles; nothing is too big or too small to qualify.

I was able to keep working throughout treatment, but cancer prompted me to use my spare time to be in stillness. In that state I could see the process of life at work and trace seemingly incongruent events coming together for good. Cancer pushes others to find unexplored endurance to keep pace with work and family demands and leaves no time for such reflection. They experience healing and a more empowered sense of self through endurance. Still others find a way to get treatment when health systems fail and it seems all may be lost. Their miracle of healing arrives through the kindness of strangers. The relationship with time, the nature of healing, and the experience of the miraculous through the treatment of cancer are different for everyone. There are no "shoulds," only "coulds."

A friend asked me what I think causes cancer. Science defines it as an uncontrolled division of abnormal cells, but this is not what she was asking. Yes, cancer cells grow too fast for the body to manage, and they end up killing themselves because they kill their host. In contemporary news coverage, social and ecological ills are often described as a cancer—they also seem to happen because we are moving too fast without regard for our host, the earth. We communicate by instant messages, gulp fast food, expect same-day delivery, and imagine we can meet our soulmate through speed dating. Instead of reading the morning paper we check our Twitter feed. Things happen in rapid succession without reflection or amends. It often seems to be spinning out of control. We do not take time to plan for the potential fallout from what we are creating. As a result we seem to be in the process of another mass extinction. The question is whether or not humans, or indeed most species, will survive it.

THE COLLAPSE OF TIME

I have no idea how to answer my friend's question, but perhaps one feature of cancer, both personal and global, is that it is a crack in the structure of time.

There are so many ways I have tried to save time. There is the urgency I have created for myself by worrying I was wasting time and thinking I had to wisely spend it. I have tried to pace myself and have been relieved when time has run out. I have fidgeted when it passes too slowly and wept when it refused to last. Life is always most precious when I simply lose track of time and become completely absorbed in what I am doing. More than any other circumstance in my life, cancer has diminished the influence of time on my choices and my capacity for radiance. For that I just might be eternally grateful.

CARDINAL MATTERS

I spent a lot of time looking out the window during the winter of my first chemotherapy. One day while I was writing, a movement in the tree at the end of the sidewalk caught my eye. This tree did not keep the seasons like others do. About a quarter of its rusty autumn leaves hung around clumps of bright red berries despite the bitter winter. It was a still day and it was odd that only the leaf that had caught my eye seemed to be moving. When I looked more closely, I saw it was a spectacular orange bird. It looked like a cardinal, but it was not red. I turned to Google and learned that indeed there are orange cardinals. Eventually it flew away and I returned to my writing. I asked several friends and no one had ever seen an orange cardinal, which made me cherish the sight of it even more, although I gave the incident no particular significance.

The following day the tree was filled with bright red cardinals, and there again was the orange one! The berries ferment when temperatures alternate between freezing and thawing, which makes the tree "party central" for birds. I had never seen so many cardinals at one time. In our language, one of the definitions of the word *cardinal* is "of the greatest importance; fundamental." If I were to look at this as a message for me, would I need to believe more in the importance of my life and surviving cancer? I had learned to think of self-importance as a character defect, but this aspect of self-importance is not about arrogance or a desire to have power over others. It is simply understanding that a life matters. What we do with it matters. It can be hard to remember this when you have been diagnosed with a life-threatening illness.

There is an interesting dance with power when you receive a dire prognosis and must suddenly make very consequential decisions. A doctor tells you the cancer is treatable, but what you will get in return for that treatment is unknowable. You try to assess information you know nothing about while taking advice from people you have just met. How do you trust yourself? How much power do you give to your doctor, to drugs, to claims for everything from frankincense to a Brazilian healer? Are you worthy of all those resources being spent on you? That question is the hardest of all to answer. It is another crack in reality, another tumble into that curious spaciousness that is divorced from the rest of your life.

Physical challenges are the most recognizable and, in some ways, the easiest to address. Life depends on meeting them, so they are the first consideration. However, it is difficult to trust your own body in even the most basic decisions once it is sick. I was nauseated from chemotherapy and having trouble even drinking water. In alternative treatments, a cancer diet might recommend things like green smoothies and raw foods and discourage things like sugar, dairy, or processed foods. I was determined to eat healthy, but raw and fresh foods made me vomit and I had not been able to stomach anything for days. I was not listening within and trusting my body's needs. Here was at least one way I was denying self-importance and giving my power away to external authorities. I finally stood in the middle of the grocery store and said to myself, "You can have anything you want." I went home with a big bag of potato

THIS DAY WON'T COME AGAIN

chips and a half gallon of chocolate milk, which went down perfectly.

A dear friend told me about her ninety-year-old mother's diet of Tootsie Rolls, Sara Lee desserts, Spice Drops, and Breyers ice cream. Her mother also took maybe three of the eight pills prescribed, whichever ones she felt like for the day, because she weighed only eighty-five pounds and thought all of those drugs were too much for her little body. She lived over a decade longer than her doctors thought possible. When my friend took her mother to the doctor, he said, "Whatever you're doing, Gracie, keep doing it because it's working." I cannot imagine this would work for anyone else, although I have joked that the long shelf life of Tootsie Rolls might have had something to do with preserving her. The point is my friend's mother listened outside *and* inside. She combined what modern medicine was giving her with her own sense of what she needed. She took advice and help without giving away her power. It is important to stress that for almost everyone, being in our power means following the course of treatment and medication outlined by our doctors. Occasionally we will get a very clear signal to honor the importance of our own body's feedback. An allergic reaction would be one example. The need to find something, anything, you can tolerate in your stomach is another.

I would not want to stop taking a new drug that makes me nauseated because it seems to be working, but I am experimenting with how to diminish the side effects. I have eliminated all sorts of things that are supposed to be healthy because they simply do not agree with me. I weigh more than I normally do, but no one on my medical team has said I need to lose weight. It is strictly my vanity, and what is vanity if not a shadow aspect of self-importance?

A lifetime of obsessing about my weight has resulted in an eating disorder. For many years it was "under control." Then

CARDINAL MATTERS

the ascites (fluid that accumulates in the body) that came with the second round of cancer caused a rapid, substantial weight gain. With chemotherapy came steroids to prevent vomiting and stimulate appetite. Following that came a drug that has to be taken on an empty stomach and causes nausea that does not go away until I eat again. The moment I am allowed, I eat with a vengeance. They tell cancer patients to eat whatever they want. They are far more concerned about weight loss than weight gain. However, many of us who suffer from irregular eating and poor body image before cancer live to be humiliated as it persists in spite of illness and treatment. I went to my family doctor to ask if they will treat an eating disorder when someone has cancer. She said she thought that made it *more* urgent, not less. Although it is devastating to have to face an eating disorder as well, cancer does not mean one cannot regain a healthy relationship with food. It also does not mean one cannot get help for issues other than cancer.

I would have thought vanity would go away because there are clearly more important things going on. But when you are bald, when your face has grown round as a full moon from steroids and your body plump as pregnancy from ascites, it is impossible not to notice people trying to keep the surprise from their faces and eyes when they see you. You recognize it because you did the same thing when talking with a woman whose face is distorted from brain-tumor surgery. Cancer has a way of inspiring a sort of dark humor that can help with the adjustment. I was talking with someone who was amazed to learn about all the hair loss. It is not only from the top of your head. You lose eyebrows, lashes, and nose hairs as well as the other clumps and meadows that normally cover your body. She asked how it grows back, what comes first. It always makes me laugh because the first hair I noticed was a longish chin hair! Redefining our worth with humor and tenderness

THIS DAY WON'T COME AGAIN

can be profoundly liberating, but there is no question it is also heartbreaking.

With all the research confirming the need to move and use our bodies in order to stay healthy, a walk or bike ride can easily become about keeping one's heart rate up, covering a certain distance, or burning enough calories. With such intentions at the root of my activity over the years I have missed much of the healing power in my environment. I have a route I like to walk, which allows me to avoid the busy streets and traffic. I tend to prefer the sunny side of each street, but one particularly warm afternoon I decided to walk in the shade. The entire time I felt like I was on the wrong street. I would have told you I was familiar with all the houses, but I could not believe how different they all seemed to me from this new perspective.

A new perspective is often an essential ingredient for healing. I derive the most benefit when I am walking not only for cardiovascular fitness but also to nurture my soul. On a beautiful evening I can slow down enough to enjoy neighbors trying to coax their golden retriever to turn the corner. He is determined to go to McDonald's, but they are headed home because that is a once-a-week treat on Fridays only. I have time for a sweet exchange with a little girl who has just learned to say hello. I meet a man who is building the addition on his home by himself. I get to thank the neighbor on whose porch I took shelter during a recent downpour. I have a lovely chat with a woman tending her garden and tell her how much I appreciate the beauty it brings to my life. I have a sense of belonging where I live as our conversations create the smiles on one another's faces. I feel the importance of life in community and not just the self-absorption with a fit body. As the possibility of a fit body is usurped by illness, one of the gifts is this willingness to slow down and be with others. In their company I remember the reason to have a body at all is to be in intimate relationship with nature, with others, and with the soul of creativity. That intimacy might not cure me, but I feel whole and radiant in the exchange of it.

Another quiet day on the sofa I felt as though countless knots in my body were being untangled and the energy locked in them was free to move again. I was losing strength and muscle tone, but I was gaining release and freedom. I decided when the time came to rebuild my strength, I would try to do it without recreating these hard, tight masses of flesh. As I stayed with the sensation it seemed that subtler, nonmuscular knots were part of the disentanglement too. Specific memories surfaced as though the beliefs that colored them and caused the emotions associated with them also were being released.

The more subtle and difficult power dances are performed at the levels of the unconscious and of spirit. I went to an appointment with my social worker thinking I had nothing to say. I could think of nothing bad, nothing good, no pivotal events or relationship issues. I silently wondered if I needed her anymore, if I should take a break. As the session bumped along and I fumbled for a topic, I mentioned I had been waking with a feeling of discomfort from difficult dreams, and that three more of my peers with ovarian cancer seemed to be taking a turn for the worse. Their progress is not mine, but when a friend dies it is as though I am on the other side of the street again. Even though the houses are all the same, everything about the way I see them has changed. The longer we live, the fewer survivors there are to keep us company. I cannot afford to give my power to the losses, but in light of them it feels irresponsible to be unprepared for my own death.

The need to embrace my own mortality brings another level of understanding to a teaching I read decades ago. It described a Buddhist spiritual practice of rising every morning and saying, "Today would be a good day to die." I thought this sounded profound and I would repeat it each morning with the belief I really meant it. About fifteen years ago, I was a passenger in a beat-up old pickup truck driving through the mountains in Mexico. The roads were winding and barely wide enough for two vehicles to meet. The driver was passing on blind curves and taking all sorts of insane risks. The truck had no seat belts, but I did not feel it would be any safer for me to get out and hitchhike. I sat back, took a deep breath, and thought, *Into your hands I commend my spirit.* He was a terrible driver but thankfully was a better intuitive. He seemed to be able to sense when there was nothing coming around the bend. Later, when we were back in the plains and driving more safely, he said I was the first person he had ever met who did not complain about his driving. He wondered why I had not said anything. I asked if it would have made any difference. He laughed and said no. After that I understood a little more clearly that I could end up in a surprising circumstance where it could well be a good day to die, and my morning declaration became a more legitimate personal practice.

Now that I have cancer the practice has deepened again. I work as though I will live and live as though I will die. Working as though I will live means there is no hurry. There will be time to do everything that needs to be done. If it does not get done, apparently it is not needed. Working as though I will live also means I need to plan for the physical future, build my business, and steward my resources. It means I must believe in my life and hold on to my visions.

Living as though I will die means I must do what is important, sometimes at the expense of what seems urgent. Like everything else, what is important varies from person to person. Cancer makes living as though I will die even more relevant and beautiful to me. It is a reminder to keep my own side of the street clean no matter what others are doing with theirs. It

CARDINAL MATTERS

is a reminder not to leave anyone in anger, and to tell people I love them while I have the chance. It is a reason to take off the wearable technology and look at the tiny flowers along the trail, to delight in the play of light and shadow through the branches. It means there is time for a story from a child or an elder, those dreamers on the bookends of life who live outside of schedules. Living under the shadow of death makes everything in this day more precious, and when we are lost in a moment, the thought of an unlived tomorrow loses some of its sting.

We all have different configurations of what matters and what can be let go of in the physical dimension of our lives. Staying in our own power and trusting our own knowing is an aspect of healing, of feeling whole and vital. We have to believe in the importance of our own preferences in order to honor them. For example, a fairly organized and orderly environment is liberating to me. I make it a priority because it gives me the clarity and confidence to move forward. It is amazing to me how many people live in chaos and have deeply meaningful, incredibly productive, creative lives. When the popular buzz was that messy people are more intelligent, I really began to question my love of order. Who knows? Perhaps a strong sense of order is a worthy compensation for a shortage of raw brilliance.

Emotions can really run off the tracks when we try to sort out what is and is not important about having cancer and the changes it brings. Some patients are angry and feel unjustly targeted. Others are filled with regret over the choices they made and the opportunities they did not live. Some cannot forgive. Many are frightened. Parents are brokenhearted over having to leave their children, and creators are tormented over their unfinished works. Feelings are not facts and they will not determine whether you live or die. They can, however, mess with whether or not you find peace and reconciliation. They can cause you to make irrational choices. They can isolate you just at the time you most need others. We might need to have our feelings, but not everyone will see it as their job to endure them. Holding everything inside might feel impossible to some while letting it all out will feel out of the question to others. As with every other aspect of our being, we have to honor our own personality and experience. There is no template that applies to everyone. We listen, watch, and learn and then pioneer our own frontier.

One of the biggest emotional knots I had to untangle was a complicated sadness over feeling like a misfit. It led to an unflattering oscillation between trying to prove I was worthy and feeling deeply ashamed of my failures and poor character. Neither extreme made for good company. In spite of this there were always people who loved me. I cherished that love, knowing it was genuine and well-intentioned, but I could not seem to feel it. It was as though they kept giving me gloves, but what I needed were shoes.

This was put into high relief when my cancer treatment ended the first time. For months I had been surrounded by people whose only goal was to help and care for me. It was as though I was finally getting those shoes I needed. I had never had this kind of attention and support where there was a clear and complete alignment between what I needed and what I received. Then I had to return to life as usual. I had to turn the wheel of each day by myself and find anew the value of my life through what I can give. Despite my gratitude for all I have received I still have to work not to return to my sadness. Not only do I want to build physical strength without recreating knots in my muscles, I also want to nurture emotional resilience liberated from habitual feelings.

Each of us has different knots to be worked through and new strengths to develop. They come from our own life stories, and the way we tell them can change as we go through the stages of healing. We can take inspiration from others, but we cannot walk in their footsteps. We must clear our own trails and build our own bridges. Attention to the unraveling of oneself through treatment ends up being a pretty rigorous version of sitting around, and doing it may seem more important than the hundred urgent demands on our time. It does not mean we will be cured, but we may live and die more liberated and peaceful, which is its own version of healing.

All day long, experiences and ideas influence us, but without quiet time to reflect and take stock, it is easy to be unaware of their impact on our system. Part of the discomfort I suffer is remembering instances where I behaved immaturely and ignorantly toward other people. These situations still make me feel ashamed. As I prattled on to my social worker, I realized I not only need to have my affairs in order but also need to release myself and others from those torturous memories. I need to be certain I have learned from the experience and that I am living differently as a result. If it is appropriate to make amends and I can find the people to whom they are owed, I must do that. If these people are no longer alive, I must make reparations in my heart and mind and move on. I must pull that energy back from self-loathing and direct it toward future loving so that I can do better.

When I get to these matters in my healing, I sometimes feel exasperated. How many times must I rework the same issues before I can be done with them? I had an insight about this process at the Guggenheim Museum. A large spiraling ramp with walls on either side goes up the center of the building. I was seeing a retrospective of an artist's work beginning with the early pieces at the bottom. At the base of the spiral you focus on the items on the walls beside you and cannot see those above. However, as you ascend through each turn of the ramp you can see the previous paintings and sculptures below. In this way you keep viewing early works in relation to later ones. By the time you reach the top of the spiral you have seen all of a life's creations in relation to one another. When I review my own life, I might seem to be reworking similar themes, but it is always from a new perspective, with different techniques and tools, with new insights into my personality and history. Everything I learn changes my relationship to the past and can be a reason to revisit it. It is a vital aspect of the art of becoming.

There is another takeaway from this analogy. Nobody lives at the top of the Guggenheim. Whatever is gained from the experience of an exhibit, you must make your way back down to the street level. All of our coming and going is through the doorway on the ground floor. In each of my life reviews there is a need to work my new understanding of the past into my present relationships and creative works. It is not enough to process it mentally, emotionally, or spiritually. I must live the healing into my very material days in sometimes large, and more often small, ways.

In quiet reflection the mind and heart can come to terms with all that is shifting. We accept that we will not go back to the way things were. We agree to go forward to the way things are becoming. The cardinals came to teach me that we do not grow less important as death draws nearer. The days become more sacred and precious not only to ourselves but to our loved ones as well. Even as our productivity dwindles and our speed diminishes, our existence is rich with purpose and meaning.

Self-importance is a character defect when used in opposition to others, but it is truly an essential basic instinct when it is a means of sustenance and actualization. I had lost the self-importance of thinking I had to accomplish certain goals or achieve a certain status for my life to have meaning or for my potential to be fulfilled. I was learning instead I needed to believe in my capacity to love. It would not be enough to be grateful for all I have been allowed to experience and learn. I also needed to believe in the worth of my using that learning to teach and mentor others. I did not have to get it all down in writing or do it for any specific audiences. I just needed to show up each day and do it with whoever came to my door. I needed to believe in the importance of my life as it is, not as I think it should be when I am well or as my culture thinks it should be when I am working at full capacity.

The mind also can be hijacked, if not by the illness itself then by the drugs used to treat it. In the world of cancer we call it chemo brain. This can be even more humbling and disturbing to self-respect than physical diminishment or emotional turmoil. Memory function goes on walkabout, names vanish into thin air, and we circle in on tasks as our mind is kidnapped by a handful of other chores along the way. Well-meaning friends joke that they have the same thing—it is called aging. However, this is not like normal aging. This is a sudden and dramatic loss that is more extreme and frightening. You fear your mental capacities will never be restored. You also talk too much, lose your train of thought, and have few if any filters. You find it hard to concentrate on what others are saying, and large gatherings are overwhelming. You might lose your ability to read and find yourself staring at a page with no memory of what is on it, though you have gone over it three times. You know you are supposed to meditate and do positive visualization, but you either fall asleep or get wound up in imaginary situations of how you will respond to complications or a miraculous remission. You have so much to decide and so little faith in your ability to do so.

Because of this, patients are advised to take support people to conferences with the doctor. They are more likely than the patient to get the facts straight and ask good questions. There is some comfort in finding that, despite the cognitive disorder, intuition and spirit remain true. They might, in fact, be more accessible because the mind is less dominant. We listen to others and learn as much as we can, but in the end, we do what "feels" right. We try to avoid what would close the door to life behind us. We go with our gut, with what brings light to our spirit, and we hope it also brings healing to our body.

The importance of resting, introspection, and integration of experience has always been part of the curriculum of the great mystical teachings. I certainly knew I was supposed to be doing it, but the culture I lived in was stressing career and the appearance of success. I have been very slow to disengage from these cultural values, but I want to trust the process of my life. It is tempting to judge it and wish it had been otherwise, but then it would not be my life. We need to be careful deciding what we want to disown. It is no better to cut out a pivotal life experience than it is to surgically remove a bladder. Both require a substitute, and the original item works best. Disentangling knots in our being is not the same as cutting them out. It is, rather, liberating the threads so the story can be rewoven into a more pliable and beautiful fabric, a more mature and artistic expression of a refining self. This is the art of healing and the importance of every person engaged in it.

It surprised me a little that some of the biggest knots I encounter in my healing process seem to have come from what I had thought was spiritual practice. It was really just an ambition to obtain what I imagined was empowerment that would surely come with being a better person. Ambition is one of my fiercest character traits. It has motivated me to learn and achieve a great deal, but it has also spilled over into jealousy, competitiveness, and self-righteousness. No wonder self-importance seemed like a serious character defect to me. Over time, as I sat in stillness and untangled one complication after another, I realized I had been afraid to surrender my ambition. I was afraid I would not be motivated to do anything and I would have nothing to give to life. However, as soon as I let go of that kind of self-importance, some more beautiful character traits began to surface. I was happy to help others succeed while I remained invisible. I was happy to sit in quiet contemplation for its own sake, rather than with the goal of being a better person. I was content to seek the sacred instead of success.

There are so many possible causes for cancer it is hard to know why one person has it and others do not. Since so many of us will have it, it makes little sense to take it personally. It is an epidemic, and why it is happening in our world at this time will be, like most of life, clearer in retrospect. Having cancer is no reason to throw God out, but neither is it a reason to get God. Miracle cures do not happen because some version of God chooses some people and not others. If there is a God, it is incomprehensible. It is hinted at in the order and radiance of life. It is sensed in miracles, sought in science, and best expressed in profound creativity. It is most appreciated in states of awe and best acknowledged by gratitude. It is approached in prayer and received in meditation. None of this is dependent on physical wellness, and none of it guarantees a cure. Healing is most exquisite when we throw ourselves at the mercy of the mystery and find ourselves in the beautiful surprises it delivers.

As I have said goodbye to my loves that died, I have noticed that by the time cancer is done with them, they seem to be ready to go. The ability to let go and accept your own life's timing is another stage of healing. What remains important is profoundly personal. If an orange cardinal or some such messenger parks outside the window or inside our awareness, we need to take note. We need to trust ourselves to learn from it no matter what state we might be in. We can reside in the truth that, as long as we receive breath, our life is wanted and beautiful.

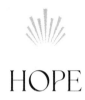

HOPE

I once heard if doctors give us a 15 percent chance of surviving, they are telling us the percentage they know about. The rest is up to us and whatever miraculous forces may be at work in our lives. There are stories about people who do little to support their own health but still outlive their prognosis, who have a complete remission and defy all the odds. Others who have taken great care and played by the rules surprise everyone by dying only weeks after being diagnosed. No matter how much time we have between diagnosis and departure, some take the possibilities they are given and live into the fullness of each day while others become paralyzed and find it challenging to embrace the life that remains for them. Most of us with cancer have a broad range of thoughts and feelings over the course of our illness and treatment. As with everything else, the way we respond to a prognosis and the possibilities we are given is personal and unique. Much depends on where we place our hope.

Some patients have religious beliefs that give structure to their hope. They personalize the source of life as a loving entity in which one may confide every thought and feeling. They share in a community committed to a way of life together and united by a common text full of wisdom and guidance. They feel supported in the wondrous but sometimes frightening universe in

HOPE

which we find ourselves. I had a very dear friend whose devout Christian faith was powerful and sustaining. One day she was telling me about the pain a tumor was causing. She said she prayed to Jesus to relieve the pain and help her sleep. She woke feeling refreshed and had no pain to start her day. As I listened, it occurred to me her prayer was not so different from the techniques for pain management another friend had been learning at a major American hospital. The most appreciable difference was that one called it visualization and credited science while the other called it prayer and thanked God. Both were grateful for the healing, and their spirits were uplifted.

Another woman I met also placed her hope in her belief in God. In her case she prayed but did nothing else to help realize her hopes. In my life, failing to take action to achieve my intentions has led to disappointment and a sense of betrayal. Whatever God may or may not be, my lesson has been that God is not a servant who simply grants my requests. I have heard it said that God cannot do for us what God cannot do through us. Seen this way, putting my hope in divine intervention is not so much making a wish list as it is a way to focus my efforts so that they are headed in a helpful direction. I do not mean to say we are not granted instantaneous miracles or that they do not sometimes come when we pray for them. However, the religious texts are not only about happy outcomes. They are also about trials and the miracles that result from doing what we must in order to meet those challenges. The stories teach us how to recognize and receive the mercy of love in the worst of circumstances.

I met another woman in the waiting room who said she knew she was going to die but it did not matter because her religion promised she was saved for all eternity. Some of us find comfort in thinking we continue on in some form after physical death, while others find that possibility terrifying. It seems we believe according to our own experiences and needs, and we find hope where we place our faith. Whatever the great creative power of the universe is, I find my hope in believing it is available to everyone, and I have learned we do not have to wait for death to know that the sacred is possible in every moment, however unremarkable it might seem at first glance.

One of my most cherished memories is of one summer evening in Ohio. I looked up into the sky and thought there was going to be a glorious sunset. I called two friends and invited them to come to Lake Erie with me. We arrived just in time to see trillions of particles scatter light rays in a passion of hot colors bleeding into blackening blue. We were delighted. I said it was wonderful, but I still missed the more brilliant reds and purples in the prairie sunsets of my childhood. One of my friends said I should sing something because my voice would carry across the water and all the people out on their boats would hear me. I said I did not know what I could possibly sing that would honor the beauty of that sky. Also, I was embarrassed and worried people would be annoyed. She kept insisting. In spite of my rebellion against religion, all I could think of was one of my father's favorite hymns. As I sang "How Great Thou Art," it was as though someone turned up the dimmer switch and the sky instantly deepened in color. It was like nothing any of us had ever seen. All along the shore people came out of their houses to listen and watch, and my friend said, "See?" I suspect science can explain what happened in that moment, but would that make the occurrence of the shift in intensity at the exact time of my singing any less meaningful? Does the fact that medicine is involved make a remission from cancer any less miraculous?

I could have asked myself just what made me think it was going to be such a great sunset and overridden the urge to go. I often do that. I could have worried about making it on time and not invited my friends, but then I would not have sung. Instead I answered the hope in each moment with a yes, and the sky delivered us a wondrous experience. Another time the sunset might have disappointed, but still I would have enjoyed homemade ice cream at Edna Mae's and the good company of friends. There are many other possible outcomes to every situation, and some, like a flat tire on the way, would be unhappy ones. If we could see beyond the immediate circumstance, we might learn the derailment of our plans put changes in motion that worked in our favor. Perhaps an accident would be avoided or we would meet someone by the side of the road who would become important to us. We are always tempted to think things would turn out best if they went according to plan, but since we cannot see into the future, we have no way of knowing. We hope for the best and meet what comes.

Whether they have religious beliefs or not, many people place their hope in the science of medicine. They actively participate in the planning of their treatment, research new therapies, and leave no stone unturned. For those who have the fire and tenacity to pursue all their options, there are sometimes powerful and positive outcomes. In other cases, there is no amount of money or effort that can change a circumstance. Some may find peace in knowing they exhausted every possibility and did not give up. For others, peace never comes, but even that can be transformed into a gift when what is learned from the experimental treatments they sign up for is used to extend the lives of future patients. No matter where we place our hope, we often need to partner it with patience, forgiveness, and surrender. These are not easy to access and practice when we have a life-threatening illness. We often need a therapist or cancer support group to help us process our experience and tap into our strengths.

There are people who put their hope in alternative medicine and healers, and with something as pervasive and pernicious as

THIS DAY WON'T COME AGAIN

cancer we need all hands on deck. For many the lack of scientific evidence or the sometimes audacious claims of these alternatives are off-putting, but people are drawn to these treatments because they have been known at least anecdotally to work. Alternatives are especially compelling when Western medicine has nothing to offer other than a terminal diagnosis. We might decide to try alternative methods first because of the toxicity and side effects of chemotherapy and radiation, and maybe we will have a remission. When we turn to Western medicine after alternative therapies fail, we still might have a remission. In less fortunate instances we might have chosen conventional treatment too late for it to work. On the other hand, we could *start* with Western medicine and turn to alternative therapies later only to discover that conventional treatments had caused irreparable damage that no alternative methods can overcome. This is where the decision-making is painfully hard. In the end we follow what gives us the most hope and must trust that, while "the choice might have been mistaken, the choosing was not." We do our best, and it is pointless to regret—it just takes the luster off a bold and beautiful rush of spirit toward life. No matter what we do, when our time has come, we all will die. The quality of our days and our capacity for wholeness no matter where we are in the trajectory of our lives are what give us joy and power.

Some people find positive visualization and meditation techniques helpful for living through the healing process, and because these approaches do not have religious overtones, they are easier for many to embrace. Some techniques have been shown in studies to have measurable benefit, while others are supported only by anecdotal evidence. Even if these methods do not cure cancer, they seem almost without fail to relieve stress, lift depression, and reduce side effects. These are invaluable supports to healing. A large measure of their benefit is in allowing one to slow down, reflect, and process treatment as it

HOPE

is happening. It can seem far less overwhelming when there is spaciousness and gentleness around invasive physical measures and the personality's responses to them. It can lead to hope in the process of one's own life even if not in the potential cure for illness. During my first round of treatments the experience of quiet reflection and contemplation was so profound I wanted never to live fast again.

When we cannot be still because of the demands of our hectic routines, our sense of purpose and the intimacy in our lives may sustain us. The love we share and the tasks we accomplish can fuel our hope. The unique conditions of our lives cause us to learn different things we then can share with one another and our caregivers to enrich our understanding and increase our collective knowledge of the healing process.

Some patients feel a tremendous responsibility for creating their own healing and leave little room for the miracles that can come through the hands of others. It is especially heartbreaking when they blame themselves and feel like failures if they do not get well. I remember having lunch with a very wise and socially active elderly couple. They were discussing the world's woes and the actions they took to counter them in an almost casual, light-hearted way. I could not help but question their good humor in the face of calamity. My hostess laughed and said, "Oh, sweetheart, we don't do things because we believe they will turn out the way we want them to. We do them because we think it's the right thing to do." Our decisions always create a full range of possibilities, and disappointment is a reasonable response to many of those outcomes. Where hope is concerned, our reaction to disappointment is as important as the circumstance itself. Do we draw irrational conclusions or become pessimistic? We want to learn from experience, but taking our lesson and making appropriate changes is different from coloring everything with an expectation of the worst. We would have many unpublished

THIS DAY WON'T COME AGAIN

best-selling novels and far fewer inventions if everyone were easily discouraged. We would also have fewer remissions. It is not always the first treatment that is the cure.

There are people who find their greatest peace in simply following directions from the experts. The less they know, the happier they are. Just tell them what to do and they will do it. They hope to get well but feel it is out of their hands. They may meet the outcome with as much or as little peace as those who have relentlessly sought to know everything possible. We have so much to learn about cancer, and an innocent kind of trust is a way many people come to their healing. It can be devastating when we place our life in the hands of people who are incompetent, careless, or just plain overworked, but in the end almost all of us place our hope in others and the treatments they provide. We rely on regulatory bodies and the guidelines they set forth. Or we rely on a supernatural order. We find our hope where we place it.

Perhaps the importance of our beliefs and strategies is not in whether or not they work but in the degree to which they allow us to have a full and vital day. Too often we become so determined to cure our cancer we put everything else on hold until we are well. We miss the opportunities for joy and fulfillment we have right now and feel betrayed when our beliefs do not deliver a cure. The capacity to live the best day possible does not depend on things going according to plan. In fact, people often find increased resourcefulness and strength in the face of extraordinary adversity, and these circumstances create outcomes beyond their wildest dreams.

One of my great teachers in living fully no matter what life delivers was a virtuoso singer from China. One day we were standing on a bridge in Italy and he said, "Life good." It was something he said many times a day, and in that moment I finally asked why. He told me his father had been killed during

HOPE

the Cultural Revolution in China, his family had been stripped of all their possessions, and they were sent to live in another part of the country. Every morning the schoolchildren had to run toward the east, toward the rising sun. One morning he complained about the blinding sun in his eyes. Because Mao Zedong was associated with the sun, my colleague was erroneously punished for complaining about the leader and was sent to prison, where he was made a cook's helper. The cook was angry with him one day and poured a vat of boiling oil on him. His body was covered with scars but he lived. Since then he says every day is a good day. At so many points he could have given up or chosen to live in fear and bitterness, but instead he became a great singer with a successful, international career. He inspires my hope when I am tempted to despair.

When we receive a difficult diagnosis and a poor prognosis, we can be so afraid of dying we find it impossible to remain concentrated and engaged in our lives. I have been questioning why there is such fear around dying, given it is inevitable, and I wonder if a great deal of it might be our unfinished business. There are broken relationships we wish we had found the means to heal, or promises we wish we had kept. Some regrets come readily to mind, and the possibility of leaving them unhealed is not easy to accept. There may be more than a few loose ends, interactions and situations that have not been resolved in ways we would have wished. We know they still have a hold on us because they cause us to blush or feel shame when we recall them. Resolving these issues is the subject of shelves worth of self-help books and programs. There would not be such an abundance of support to heal the past as one nears the end of life if it were not such a common and important desire. It might not be prudent to engage in a reconciliation process with the past in the hope to be cured, but the desire to be at peace with oneself and others while there is still time can lead to incredible healing. It can help us become more at ease with both living and dying. It can give us hope that we at least may heal our misdeeds if not our disease.

The only reason to treat cancer is for the lives we hope to have. If we lose our liveliness in the process, there is no gain and possibly even greater loss. Each and every day is so ripe with possibility we can never take advantage of a fraction of it. To avail ourselves of nothing but despair and anxiety will not necessarily keep us from being cured, but neither does it contribute to our healing. It does not give us the freedom and vitality to live into our gifts and share our love. To live into the mystery of life is to trust the unfolding of our own process. What comes is ours to do, and what we create around it is ours to choose. There are certainly many actions we can take to participate in our wellness, from diet and exercise to emotional intelligence and spiritual practice. Having purpose and meaningful relationships also seem to be significant factors in our healing. However, it does not matter in what entity we place our hope—cancer eventually calls our beliefs and choices into question. This is one of its gifts, so to speak.

When we are not living down or up to arbitrary odds in a prognosis, we can live into the moment knowing it will never come again. Perhaps we can actually carve out the time to take that bike ride or go to the beach. Maybe we can pinch even a couple minutes to send a text if we cannot make the phone call. What if we risk starting an improbable project and discover it actually pays more than the work that has been robbing our vitality?

Hope can be found in the tiniest of actions. There is hope in putting on makeup and getting dressed for a day that could be miserable, if the way we are feeling at present is any indication. It is an affirmation that we are available for goodness and beauty to abide alongside the challenges. Maybe we cannot take the time for even one more small thing because of others depending

HOPE

on us, but maybe we can live into our hope by being willing to believe that at some point in the future we might yet find a way. What does not cure us, or succeed as we had imagined, may yet fulfill our hope to contribute meaningfully to the future.

Hope can grow in every heart. It is where we begin and end, and it is as constant as the polestar as we navigate our passage through life. It sharpens our senses. It helps us to mind the details, to listen for what is between the lines, to ask for a second or third opinion. It inspires us to stretch beyond the scope of our own lives, to draw courage from the adventures others have dared, and to try for the sake of future generations.

Cancer drags us back and forth through the entire territory of our personality. It takes courage to face the questions that arise. Should we risk stopping the demanding job in order to heal the family, or could we risk asking the family to take greater responsibility for themselves so we can secure our legacy at work? Sometimes others celebrate the changes we make, not only because they are genuinely happy for us but also because they are happy for what they achieved themselves when they no longer relied on us. Solutions often arise that we could not have foreseen. Circumstances have a way of resolving our concerns in ways we could not have dreamed, if we allow them to. There is never a guarantee the choices we make will pan out, but there is always reason to hope.

A valid inquiry is: Are we using our approach to healing as an attempt to control the outcome or as a means to investigate the intense mystery in which we find ourselves? Decisions can seem so vitally important, but without being able to see into the future, it is impossible to know what is best. Still, we must choose something and make a day of it. Life is not a problem to be solved—it is a mystery to be lived. A great part of healing is overcoming the anxiety of impermanence and the insecurity of life. Perhaps we love daredevils because they live into the danger and show us it can be done. I have often heard great risk takers being described with admiration because they died doing what they loved. Hope is the wind in the sails that carries a ship out of a safe harbor to fulfill its daring purpose at sea.

We need hope not only to heal from cancer but also to confront the numerous, gnarly problems in our world. We cannot know exactly how we will solve the issues of climate change, racism, famine, oppression, and epidemics, but we continue to work at them because we have hope in our humanity and creativity to triumph over fear and scarcity. As each of us moves one little bit forward in the places where we have energy and resources to assert ourselves, the whole of our collective humanity is moved. I think of the drops of water in the Colorado River forming the Grand Canyon over a period of twenty million years. A single drop might not have much of an impact, but countless drops working together over eons can. The challenge is to sustain the hope that a larger possibility is created by our individual actions. Hope has a way of bringing us to our causes and the good we might do. For those of us with cancer, healing in the face of this disease that has become an epidemic often becomes the cause we choose.

Hope is a double-edged sword. By definition it is a feeling of expectation or desire for a certain outcome, but it can lead to heartbreak when we treat it as a certainty rather than a possibility. Hope is not built for predicting outcomes, only for moving us toward them. Some of us will need to let go of hope in order to find our peace, while others will experience joy in sustaining hope through their last breath. Hope can seem absurd in the face of death, but we all know the stories of people who return from a coma and live into a sensational shift of consciousness that inspires the world. Too often hope begets disappointment and discouragement, but without it there is little reason to get out of bed in the morning. The challenge is to navigate between

HOPE

hope and despair while embracing the inevitable mystery that is life. Hope can keep you up at night thinking about how to achieve your goals. It can illuminate your dreams and speak through the most unexpected people. It can jump off a billboard or fall off a shelf. It will try everything at hand and it will never stop trying. Hopelessness is for people who don't read the fine print. There we find a caveat reminding us not to quit before the miracle.

ABIDE WITH ME

When loved ones learn we are facing a life-threatening illness, some of them flood our inboxes with links, articles, and offers to help. Others show up at our homes with stuff. They are worried, maybe awkward, maybe hoping to cheer us up. Some do the opposite—they stay away thinking they will give us our privacy and allow us to rest. Their intention, one way or another, is to do for us what they think they would want for themselves. They are practicing the Golden Rule: to love others as you love yourself. It is probably the most universal relationship advice ever given. It sounds good, not too complicated.

The trouble is one person's favorite comfort food might be something another person cannot stomach. Some people like to be distracted in times of trouble, while others like to focus on the issues to try to find clarity. Some really do like to hunker down in solitude. Some people like to receive advice and follow another's lead, while some feel bullied by too much input. The Golden Rule is not designed to work at the level of the personality where we try to do for others what we like to do for ourselves. The Golden Rule does work, but it is not a teaching directed only at the personality of the caregiver. It is aimed at the souls of both the caregiver and the recipient. The relationship between someone who is ill and a caregiver can be rich and beautiful. It can also be uniquely challenging. It is like an improvisational dance in which each learns to anticipate the other's moves in order to interact gracefully, with harmony and rhythmic synchronicity.

The soul does not listen the same way as the personality. It does not care about the same things, and it has a different set of filters. It does not hear that you should love others by sharing the things you like to have yourself. And it does not hear that you should love others *before* or *after* you love yourself. It does not consider for even a moment that you could love anybody *more* than you love yourself. The soul hears what it really means to "love others *as* you love yourself." To the soul, the Golden Rule is saying, "Right here, right now, whatever shape you're in, see if you have any capacity for love and *be* that capacity." It is not a suggestion for a horizontal exchange of niceties. It is a call to a vertical alignment with love. When love talks to the soul, it is like a bell with a feather tongue, like a harp with silk strings. It is quieter than ideas. It is more tender than touch. It travels past prayers to claim the miracles that have already taken place before we even ask for them. From an old story written back in the sixth century BCE, we learn something about how the soul responds to the Golden Rule with inspired friendship:

> When Job's three friends heard of all this evil that had come upon him, they made an appointment to come together to show him sympathy and to comfort him. And when they saw him from a distance, they didn't recognize him. And they raised their voices and wept, and they tore their robes and sprinkled dust on their heads toward heaven. And they sat with him on the ground seven days and seven nights, and no one spoke a word to him, for they saw that his suffering was very great.

I called my mother once when I was feeling frayed and crooked. I was trying really hard to be brave because I did not want her to worry, but my voice cracked and the tears were not far behind. She did the most perfect thing. She sat on the other end of the phone and cried with me. She had never done that before and she never did it again. In that moment it was exactly what I needed, but it probably would not have worked another time. It was not a recipe—it was grace.

In practice, at the level of the personality, expressing love can mean a thousand things. We have to be ready for anything, and we have to be ready for nothing. We have to learn how to show up for each other as if we have never met, even though we might have years, sometimes a lifetime, of history together. Everything about relationships changes around illness because we are suddenly thrust into a deeper sense of the sacredness and preciousness of life. However, the response to that awareness is not universal. Some of us will shift into overdrive, trying to complete everything that remains undone. Others will want to drop all the doing and get still. It gets complicated when the patient is a doer and the caregiver thinks they need to be still, or when the patient has dropped into reflection and quietude and their partner thinks they need to get off the couch. Neither is wrong. It is just that sometimes we end up caring about things that do not matter to one another.

Sometimes a healing crisis draws us closer to our loves. The strong relationship we have built endures the storm. Sometimes there is even a stunning new flowering of our love. In other cases, the weakness of a relationship snaps and we abandon one another just when our need is greatest. Sometimes the kindness of strangers turns into new and sustaining loves. Most of us find we have a broad experience that includes the whole spectrum of possibilities. It can seem like salt in the wound for both patients and caregivers to have to deal with relationship issues on top of everything else, but there is no way around it. We want mighty companions to move forward with us. We do not want to feel alone with what we are learning, but we cannot hold hands if we cannot walk at the same pace. A friend came to visit when I was in the middle of chemotherapy. I took her to see Niagara Falls. She was so excited she bolted ahead at her New York City pace, which is a street version of speed walking. There was nothing I could do to match her pace. I simply did not have the strength. If two people want to walk side by side, the stronger one must slow down. The same is true of emotional, mental, and spiritual realities: the one with the most capacity has to accommodate the other.

Sometimes we get into trouble because we assume all the need is in the person with the illness, and we imagine those around them should do all the adjusting. In terms of physical capacity this might be true. However, experiencing one's worth and potency is part of the healing process. When we are trying to heal, it does not matter if we are exhausted, bald, missing body parts, or wheeling a medication tree alongside us. Most of us still want to be in the world and engaged in our relationships, spontaneously and consciously if we can. This is life now. We want to work at the changes that are forcing their way into our relationships. Our being ill does not let us off the hook. If we decide a change is in order, no matter how we are feeling, we must own our power and take the initiative.

When trying to give care, it is important to see loved ones as whole people, not just as their disease. When tempted to give unsolicited advice, it is helpful to understand it might land as criticism. When caregivers are overprotective or hovering, those suffering illness might feel infantilized. Then again, some people who are ill want to be waited on. They want all the decisions made for them. Together both patient and supporter have to come to an agreement about what is fair and empowering to everyone involved. On both sides of the equation, it is merciful to remember that, even when there is deep gratitude for life itself, there can still be grief for what has been lost. Either patients or their loved ones may feel transformed by an illness. Both may feel betrayed by it. Some may become angry, others depressed. Some may feel hopeless, and some may be in denial. People with life-threatening illnesses and their caregivers feel different things at different times and in no specific order. No one knows how they will respond until they are in it, and once they are in it, it is not worth trying to be anything except true to oneself.

Navigating relationships through the process of healing is sometimes confusing because love has different frequencies, which are identified with qualities like sympathy, empathy, or compassion. Sometimes the personality gets stuck in one or another frequency, and if it is not what is needed it can be frustrating.

Let us imagine two people are in a car driving down the street. There is another car in front of them and, a little farther ahead, a friend is walking their dog. The dog gets loose, runs into the street, and is hit by the first car.

In the frequency of *sympathy*, the passenger in the second car runs to the dog owner and says, "Oh, my dear, I'm so sorry for you. What a tragic thing to have your dog run over by a car."

In the frequency of *empathy*, the passenger in the second car runs to the dog owner and says, "Oh, I know how you must feel. My dog was run over last year and it was heartbreaking."

In the frequency of *compassion*, the passenger in the second car runs to the dog to see if there is anything that can be done to help it.

All three frequencies are wonderful and important. Compassion for the dog itself is most needed at the moment of the collision. However, it would not be useful to talk about what should have been done at the scene of the accident when you are helping your friend bury the dog. That is the time for sympathy. Two months later, when the friend is having difficulty adjusting to life without the dog, is the time for empathy.

There are more than three frequencies of love. The point is the soul operates outside of time and habit, so it has a better chance of partnering with spirit to match frequencies and make the most graceful impact in each circumstance.

Spirit is a universal force, the truth of which remains constant. It permeates life, is consistently available to everyone in equal measure, and does not prefer anyone over another. It fuels human inspiration and creativity in the same way oxygen sustains the body. Spirit can reveal insights that have not been learned from life experience. It might be received as intuition or interpreted as a sudden flash of understanding.

The soul is an individual formation. We each have our own unique soul that nurtures what is within our being and directs our life force into the world. It is that part of us that can hear spirit's message and translate it into actions that are perfectly matched to the needs of the moment. It can move us to respond appropriately without pause. There is no formula for this, and spirit and soul do not care what state the personality is in. Fear is okay. Rage is okay. Every state is a perfect state from which to act with grace. In the moment when we turn everything over and say, "Help me," the soul and spirit work things out faster than we can think at the level of the personality. The soul does not need to know or like someone to feel compelled to help. In fact, sometimes strangers do better because they have no agenda for us and we have none for them. In an inspired moment we are not limited to what we have learned in the past. We outstrip the plans we made to be good and positive in the future. In such a moment we serve the very creative force of our lives.

We can prepare the soul to be at the ready to serve spirit's messages. We can listen for that still, quiet voice in the early morning, before the shutters fly open within the crazed cities of our minds. We can return in the evening to surrender our demons and forget ourselves, knowing the grace of healing is "near to the brokenhearted and saves the crushed in spirit." We can turn to the still center of our unknowable source and attend to practices like prayer or meditation. We can read inspired literature and share the promises it holds. I have found assurances for the power of love in every faith tradition I have explored as well as in secular writings. Some from my Christian upbringing are always with me. The personality doubts such things, but the soul flies to the promise of love like a moth to a flame. It becomes the wick and burns with the glory of love that ignites us and creates of us a light. Where the personality surrenders, the ecstasy of love begins.

As time goes on and the body recovers, survivors start to look normal and loved ones return to their own busy lives. Beneath the surface survivors are haunted by what has happened to them and the knowledge that it can start again at any moment. In the physical world there are lingering side effects that will not let them forget. The scars have healed, but they still feel the missing parts of their bodies. A loved one's care is not a substitute for a working bladder. Because of neuropathy, precious things slip from tingling hands and shatter cherished memories. Lips grow numb in the cold and words become slurred as if one is drunk and pretending to be sober. Brains freeze and the resulting confusion is frustrating to everyone. Reading is a delight of the past. Survivors are grateful that others love them no matter what, but that does not mean it is not heartbreaking to no longer have a reliable mind. It is just as heartbreaking for loved ones to live with someone who is so changed.

Cancer survivors bury dear friends whose treatment, the same as theirs, was not successful. They want to live for those who have loved them faithfully, who love them still, but they realize others grow weary of the complaints as much as they themselves grow weary of the treatments. When one has cancer, it can be hard to remember the body is a temple for the soul and that a life's purpose is greater than one's doings. It is hard to lose capacity in the world and deepen in spirit. It is hard to surrender to the process of life with illness and still see oneself as good and acceptable and perfect. Remembering all of this is just as challenging for caregivers and loved ones as it is for those with illness.

As the evolution of healing and relationships continues, so does the unpredictability. Sometimes patients are swept up in gratitude and a determination to live a life of joyful service. They are an inspiration. Sometimes survivors need to ignore illness and live as though it never happened. They are a mystery. Sometimes people with a life-threatening illness need to talk about it. They are companions for fellow survivors. Sometimes survivors are grateful. They are a gift. Sometimes they have trouble forgiving life for what it asks of them. That is when it can be helpful to feast on those promises in inspirational texts, whether one believes in them or not. Just as it is necessary to keep eating through nausea and loss of the sense of taste, it is essential to keep seeking and practicing good mental and emotional habits through heartbreak and the revision of everything that could once be taken for granted. These practices can be nurturing even when one does not feel like doing them.

No matter where we are in the progress of healing, whether we are survivors or supporters, we need our relationships and we need them to be growing in their capacity for love. "Two are better than one, for if they fall, one will lift up his fellow. If two lie together, they keep warm. And though a misfortune might prevail against one who is alone, two will withstand it." This is what the soul hears when we turn heavenward, as Job's friends did, seeking the love that will enable the personality to serve others even *as* it serves itself. This is what my mother did on the other end of the phone.

Cancer comes to have a relationship with everyone who is affected by it, and if we do not listen to it, we cannot learn from it. It speaks a different frequency from the rest of our being. Much of the medicine and healing is in the story we tell about the experience we are having, and it is not one-size-fits-all. Some of us have to forgive, some have to set boundaries. Some have to work less. Some need to share more. Some need to have gratitude, while others must learn to receive. Change is never easy, and the changes that come with life-threatening illness can be dramatic and more disruptive than usual. This is as true for caregivers as it is for those who are ill. The simple truth is not all relationships will survive it, and sometimes it is the closest ones that fall apart.

I had always found it easy to be an advocate for my students but was woefully inept at standing up for myself. It is a devilish issue when we have cancer. The importance of our treatment is uppermost, but what is the point of getting well if everything else is compromised in the process? We need not only our work and our relationships but also our self-reliance and integrity. We might find we are unwilling now to do some of the things we believed we had to do in the past to keep our lives running smoothly. As we untie these knots of obligation, those around us might find our new perspective untenable. We might have believed we could not live without these relationships and might be about to learn we cannot live with them.

Death of a loved one stretches relationship beyond the bounds of time and place, while the loving heart journeys a little with the one who dies. It is as though our physical world is redefined because our beloved's spirit, liberated from the body, is so expansive. Memory flutters through decades like a butterfly in a garden fully abloom. The past and the present are engulfed by eternity, and the light is so bright it washes all the colors into white. From this perspective we somehow keep breathing and life expresses its will to go on. This tear in the fabric of days will mend, but it will mean something different now to be whole. As the world changes, it is natural to fuss a while about what is being lost, but eventually we must focus on what is being called. We never can go back. This stage of life must also be spent, and we are the ones who must do it. We have to get our brains taxed, our hearts broken, and our hands dirty. Both life and death exist. Neither is deserved. Each is given.

The challenge to our relationships is not only death itself but also the way its coming hangs over everything and has us living our days in its shadow. It takes a great awareness to embrace it openly when necessary and to put it aside when possible. There are a lot of reasons why people find it difficult to talk about death, not the least of which is superstition. There is a sort of magical thinking that if we accept death as a possibility, we will create it as a probability. My father thought he was dying for the last fifteen years of his life and never missed an opportunity to let us know. His declaration and preoccupation with death seemed to have no effect whatsoever on his physical health. When, at the age of eighty-nine, he actually *was* dying, it took us a while to take it seriously. We can talk about it or not, but many who have felt they could not broach the subject of death do not get to say proper goodbyes or heal the raw scrapes and bruises of their relationships.

It is difficult when people in a relationship are not at the same stage of engagement with the inevitability of death. As with so many other matters, the one who is most able must take the lead, and sometimes must do it alone. When the most capable person happens to be the one who is dying, their loved ones are surprised to find everything has been handled. Every closet has been cleaned, the funeral service is written, and the accounting is done. That mysterious look and gentle smile may have meant a hundred things to others, but those who were dying were taking a long sip of pleasure under a breathtaking sky. If we allow it, this may be the most grace-filled, exquisite exchange of intimacy we could ever know. Enlightened death is a beautiful thing. If those of us left behind do not recognize it at the time, it may later grow on us and peace will come when we are ready.

If the greater ease is with caregivers or loved ones and not with those dying, there still is no need to impose one's reality on the other. There are as many ways to die as there are ways to live, and people will do it according to their own personality and circumstances. If neither person in a relationship can deal with the impending reality of death, there might be a truckload of unfinished business, but still there is no need to despair. There is no scenario at the end of which we cannot find peace and reconciliation. Our personalities may be limited, but love is not. The support of grief counselors and spiritual mentors can be very helpful in healing our disrupted relationships.

As much as it can be difficult to navigate existing relationships when we are in a healing process with a life-threatening illness, it can also be difficult to begin new ones. Some of us might find it exhilarating, but others will not have the energy to start at the beginning with someone. Some of us will feel it is unfair to involve someone in our lives when we are so close to the end. We might stop enjoying anything new, feeling that it is somehow wasteful or unnecessary. I noticed I had stopped buying new clothes or getting things for my home. I would see something I liked but decide I should wait until I am well to invest in it. One day, shortly before Christmas, I went to the closet to find something to wear and ended up in tears. Nothing fit properly anymore, and even if I could get it on, it seemed dull and unattractive. I threw on my father's old flannel bathrobe and went to the kitchen to make coffee. While checking email I saw a message from someone I had only recently met saying she wanted to take me to lunch and buy something new for me to wear for Christmas. She is a gifted intuitive, but you have to admit that was fast! I would not normally accept such a gift from someone I had just met, but I received another kind of healing because I embraced my new friend's generosity. It opened me to the unexpected blessings relationship can bring when I am able to receive. When I prayed for a miracle the morning I realized I had cancer, I had no idea how many forms miracles could take and how they could unfold in one surprise after another.

If every day is a good day to die, any day could also be a good day for a new dress or maybe even a new friend. There is no right time to play small with ourselves or with others. Showing up for my relationships means showing up in my creative best. It is the way I invite others to engage with me as someone who is living and not as someone who is dying. Clothes just happen to be one of my media, but they will not be important to everyone. Each of us will have our passions and ways of expressing our vitality. However close we might be to dying, we need to believe in our living. I heard about a woman who was weeping for the poignant joy of starting to read again. It had always been her great passion, but she had given it up thinking there was no point. There is always a point! The brilliance of our creative expression need not be diminished by the prognosis of our disease.

All of these things we do are what we bring to life and to one another. To have healthy, vital relationships throughout and after treatment, we need to stay engaged with our passion. It might have us doing the things we have always loved, or we might be embarking on new adventures, but nothing is more draining than falling into a rut of fear, complaints, or

THIS DAY WON'T COME AGAIN

hopelessness. Although my body is less excited to be moving, my mind less likely to dream, and my heart less inclined to hope, these changes are not the downer I had imagined they would be. As I engage in the art of first gear, there is an emerging steadiness. It is a gentler pace ripe with sensuality and peculiar details.

Some of these surprising days open like a wrinkled page from childhood history I decided not to discard. An old friend calls and I thank my lucky stars that others on that page, family and friends, are choosing to populate sentences yet to be written. Other days are purposefully folded around unshared secrets. They are letters I wish I had never opened, but they can never be unread. Some days the page is empty. It is a quiet spell bigger than punctuation and inviting pause. Some days are justified and ready for publishing while others have scribbling in the margins, portions highlighted for do-over with arrows and symbols suggesting how the details should move to create more healing. The stories we share, every page and every stage, are part of the healing that takes place between the introduction of cancer and the epilogue. Being in relationships means reading the whole book, including the topics suggested for discussion. You do not need a degree to be literate in the language of love. Kind eyes and kneeling hearts do not need an interpreter. They turn the page and read with you in the remaining light.

GENERATIVE CONVERSATION

I turned myself inside out trying to make a special time for us. She constantly criticized me and complained about the accommodations and restaurants I had arranged. I felt she was impatient, demanding, and inconsiderate of everyone around us. I quietly asked her to notice others. She felt attacked, and she was not wrong. I was now criticizing her. In one heartbroken moment I decided I did not care if our decades-long friendship ended. I raised my voice. She responded by telling me she was perfect and I was the problem. I asked her to leave. She refused. I endured the remainder of her stay, but I was never so happy to see the backside of another person. I was bald, nauseous, weak, and exhausted. I had no idea how long I had to live, and this was not how I had imagined things would go with the person who I had thought was one of my dearest and best friends.

It was not my friend's fault, nor was it mine. Neither of us had any idea how cancer would come between us and change the way we had always been together. Nothing in our past could have prepared us for it. In my life I have learned that new circumstances interrupt the flow I am in and force me to learn lessons I would never ask for or wish on anyone else. My friend and I eventually reconciled our cherished friendship, but not until time and silence had done their work.

In the stories patients have shared with me, I have learned I am not the only one who has felt disappointed and hurt, who was completely unprepared for the questions and conversations that need to happen. When you are newly diagnosed with cancer, an important decision is whom you will tell, whom you will protect, and from whom you will protect yourself. There are questions and conversations that could help us learn things we need to know about each other in order to make those decisions.

Some of us will be especially private about having cancer, wanting neither pity nor advice, and almost no one will know about our condition. Others will be very open and have tremendous ease with any and all conversation about illness. Some will welcome suggestions and hear them as love being expressed rather than feeling criticized or bossed. Others will feel judged or bullied. If we tend to work things out through conversation and do not have supportive people we can speak with, it may be very difficult for us. Others may believe talking about cancer gives it power or means we are not brave. This may frustrate caregivers who are looking for cues for how they might best support the one who is ill. Indeed, not being able to talk about anything *but* cancer can make us a burden to be endured. On the other end of the spectrum, people might encourage us to speak about it, because of their compassion or curiosity, and we might think it is none of their business.

Although talk of a certain kind can create conflict, talking generatively can prevent misunderstanding and open us to the resources of others. It is important not to assume we know how the other person is feeling or what they need. If we have a thought such as, *This must be frustrating for you*, we can ask, "How is this impacting you?" In this way we do not impose our assumptions or opinions on others. We give them an opportunity

GENERATIVE CONVERSATION

to share their experience with us, and then we can respond with empathy and compassion. When people speak from curiosity rather than from past experience, new ideas and understanding emerge that can surprise both parties.

Open conversations between patients can be practical and mundane, sharing tips for navigating treatment and living with cancer. We learn practical things like the benefits of timing medications in order to function better at work. If we are thirsty but get nauseated drinking water, a friend might suggest sucking on ice. We share recipes for high-energy foods that are easy on the digestive system. We all have different jewels of wisdom that improve the quality of our days. Talking in a generative manner is different than complaining. We are informing, or discussing in the hopes of learning, or sometimes simply easing the burden of solitude. Then again, sometimes we need to complain because, the truth is, cancer can be unbearable.

Much of our conversation is not about the disease itself but about all that comes with it. The physical side effects may dominate at first: nausea, fatigue, and neuropathy. Cancer can be hard to escape because these lingering side effects never let you forget. Then when you finish treatment, every twinge and twitch is a potential symptom of its return. Dealing with these after effects is especially challenging when the type of cancer you have does not produce particularly distinguishable symptoms. Sometimes our conversations put one another at ease, and sometimes we encourage one another to talk to our oncologist to get more informed advice. We are not always our own best friends when it comes to assessing what is going on and what to do about it. I once heard a fellow say his mind was a darkroom where he developed negatives.

It is sometimes true that keeping things to ourselves can make it worse. At the same time, if we tell the wrong person, we can set ourselves up for bad advice or painful experiences

THIS DAY WON'T COME AGAIN

like the one I had with my friend. We need to learn how to deal with emotional swings as well as side effects and encourage one another to get the right kind of help from the right person when we need it. As I often say, do not go to the hardware store if you need milk.

Generative conversation can be helpful when we are trying to understand what we believe about cancer and how that belief is working for or against us. If we equate cancer with death, it can make going through treatment seem futile and frightening. It can make us less appreciative of our caregivers, less responsive in relationships, and less creative in our work. There is a good possibility we are too much in our illness and not enough in our lives. Generative conversation can renew our relationships and draw us back into our sense of purpose. Cancer might not allow us to hope for a length of days, but it need not rob us of this day's promise. It need not make us ungrateful or self-protecting. All the good we can think and extend may not give us more time, but it can give us the time we have.

In and of itself death is a neutral event. It is an inevitable part of life. However, our beliefs and the conversations we have about it turn it into all sorts of things, from tragedy to liberation. That we as a culture talk so little about it is part of the reason it holds so much power over us. I have heard my elderly relatives and friends say they would like to pass peacefully in their sleep or surrounded by loved ones. They would prefer not to deteriorate cell by cell into increasing states of dysfunction. The fear might not be of death itself but rather of the manner of dying.

One of the hardest things to understand about death is why it comes too soon to some and leaves others lingering for too long. How is a life glorified by being cut short or dragged through suffering? It is another of the deep mysteries of time. Most of us aim to be comfortable in life, yet every day we are

GENERATIVE CONVERSATION

called upon to learn something new, which more often than not is *un*comfortable. The expected does not generate learning or carry us the next step into our collective evolution. We must learn not only as individuals but also as communities, and for both we need the unforeseeable along with communication about it once it occurs. The art of evolutionary learning is to remain curious, flexible, and creative. Diminishing states of health do not necessarily disable all our capacities. They often lead to increasing reserves of courage and humor. I was fortunate to hear spiritual teacher Ram Dass speak near the end of his life about all he has experienced since a debilitating stroke. He referred to his body as "this ick" and in the same breath spoke radiantly about the love sustaining him.

We all can have this radiant quality of life and a sense of purpose at any stage of an illness, even though we would not have believed it possible until we are living it. However, in order to experience this, we might have to change our frame of reference. A generative conversation is often the doorway through which we make this kind of shift. I remember my parents telling me it was tiring to be with friends who complained all the time about declining physical abilities. They told me they decided they would talk instead with gratitude about all the things they still could do. I realized how they were living into that practice while climbing the stairs behind my father near the end of his life. He was placing his fists on steps above him and using the strength of his arms to compensate for his failing knees. At the top he turned and looked down at me with a huge grin and said, "I can still do the stairs." My parents adopted an approach to the changes in their abilities that gave them happier days and made them more fun to be with.

Feelings are perhaps the most popular focus of our healing conversations. Unlike the body or thoughts, feelings are unstructured, amorphous. Trying to pin them down can be like

THIS DAY WON'T COME AGAIN

trying to lasso clouds. And there are so many of them! We were always asked about anxiety and depression when we checked in for our chemotherapy appointments, but feelings, whether in or out of treatment, are not so black-and-white. There are many shades of emotion. We can be irritable without going all the way to anxious; we can be weepy without being depressed. Conversation can restore us to a sense of humor. This does not mean we are a laugh a minute, but rather we can look at the lighter, glass-half-full side of things. Our hope is restored in the process of life, even if not in the likelihood life will be prolonged.

One of the hardest feelings for people diagnosed with cancer is of being isolated. We know we are not alone or unloved, but we are alone with the possibility of our own mortality. It is hard for someone to get inside that bubble with us. Other cancer patients have a better understanding, but even within our demographic we all experience our illness and prognosis differently. It can even be harder to rely on other cancer patients to be our companions because there is so much death in our community. Being face-to-face with death on a continual basis works for some of us—in learning how to die, we learn how to truly live as a result. For others it is too painful or raw and it makes things worse. Having an ongoing conversation with a qualified therapist or spiritual counselor who is experienced in supporting people with life-threatening and terminal illnesses can be the best mode of healing our relationship with thoughts about death. Whatever way we choose to go about it, dealing with feelings takes as long as it takes, and many of us need someone with us before we can do that work.

The problem for those of us who need to move all the way through the fear, anger, and sadness of our prognosis before we can begin to make peace with our situation is that we grow weary with ourselves or others grow weary with us before we get there. We try to talk ourselves out of our feelings, or others try

GENERATIVE CONVERSATION

to talk us out of them, and the pressure to be okay can be as bad as, if not worse than, the original feelings. We might resort to all sorts of compensatory behaviors trying to mitigate our emotions or to distract ourselves from the discomfort. We may not feel better until we finally give in and feel it all. It is pure grace when there is someone to go through the pain with us, whether it is our loved ones, fellow patients, or trained professionals. In the territory of our broken hearts, we do not need people to fix us. That makes us feel unacceptable and inadequate. We need them to be *with* us. That helps us believe we will make it through. Their comfort, empathy, and willingness to learn along with us are the greatest gifts we can receive.

I did not learn how to swim until I was in my forties. Diving into water was terrifying to me, so my instructor and I started out with me sitting on the side of the pool. I was to put my hands and arms in a triangular shape above my head and fall headfirst into the water. The instructor said I could go whenever I was ready. I knew I would never be ready, but I trusted her to save me, so I decided to count to three and go. It was thrilling, a total rush. I swam back to the edge of the pool anxious to do it again and was amazed to find I was just as afraid the second time. I still have to count to three when I want to dive headfirst into water.

Diving into a conversation about spirituality and what, if anything, it might have to do with death or living can feel perilous too. For many, spirituality is an intensely personal matter and not something to discuss with anyone. For others there is an intense need to engage in the conversation. By definition, God does not exist for atheists, but spirituality might. Learning to talk about spirituality without using the word *God* can be generative for all of us. For those who believe in spirituality there is such a diversity of ideas that we need to listen deeply and take great care with our own biases and language in our conversations. One woman who was an agnostic said on her deathbed, "This could be interesting." I love that in that moment she was willing to not know. She embraced the possibility of the human spirit continuing on into the adventure of death, and she accepted the possibility of nothing.

Much of my life I did not want to live. Even though I was turned against religion by early experience, it was my hope of a spiritual dimension to our humanity that kept me moving forward every day. The inexplicable phenomena and synchronicities of my unpredictable life sustained my curiosity and kept me seeking. Also, wise and charismatic people better at wrestling with life-and-death issues have kept me intrigued and optimistic.

Shortly after I decided it was time to give up on my singing career, I saw a picture of a woman in a catalogue from a retreat center. I immediately thought I needed to work with her and signed up without understanding anything about what she did. It turned out to be one of the most pivotal experiences of my life. The first thing we were asked to do was to write on a large green heart why we had come. We then walked around the room in silence and read one another's hearts. I had written, "I want to want to live." My father had always said he was putting the fear of God into us. He believed that was his duty. During that retreat I decided I did not want the fear of God in me; I wanted the *love* of God. Seeking love was a much more generative approach to spirituality, and it fueled my desire to live. The teacher's highly developed skill and techniques helped me to reach deep inside myself and connect with that passionate desire. I really did want to live, but certain beliefs and habits would have to die in order for me to do it joyously.

One of the great learnings of my life is that when it feels like I need to die, it is only that some concept I am carrying or

GENERATIVE CONVERSATION

cherishing needs to die. It might be a belief, a fear, or a dream. One by one, the attempts to manage the insecurity of life have needed to fall away, and I have had to stumble through the chaos by growing in ways I never would have signed up for. It can be easier to do that growing when we have generative conversations with others who have language and compassion that empower us rather than make us feel wrong.

I went to a wonderful lecture by a Japanese philosopher whose name, I am sorry to say, I cannot recall. However, I shall always remember him saying he had wanted to kill himself until he realized you do not die anyway. He said if the well-known teaching that "all are one" is true, it makes no sense to want our life to be other than what it is. It is best to live the life we are having with humility and gratitude. Spirituality for this man was expressed in the interconnectedness of all things. This is what I perceive as the energy grid. Although it has been years since I heard him speak, the longer I live the more I relate to his views. It has been a long time since I have wanted anything other than the one precious life I have.

For many, spiritual beliefs are rooted in a religion and a built-in community of like-minded people. They engage in generative conversations informed by shared convictions, and they learn together. Others do not identify with any religion at all but do believe in spirituality and expansive states of mind. It also is generative to discover that prayer or meditation are not the only practices that draw us into presence and expansive awareness. Almost any kind of devoted, regular activity such as sports, arts, or gardening can focus our attention and invite inspiration. Whenever people are dedicated to a common endeavor or share in generative ways with others, they seem not to be thrown so far off course by illness. However, there is no panacea. With or without religion or other anchoring practices, we can feel lost at sea and fear there will never again be solid ground to stand on. When I stumble upon someone with the exceptional capacity to receive a difficult diagnosis or face death and say, "Well, this could be interesting," I count it a blessing and try to learn from them.

Looking death in the eyes can be a head-on collision with the limits of our human understanding. Some of us who have seriously considered taking our own lives have lived along this boundary before. We have needed to search for reasons to keep going. Others have been able to take life in stride, living in very practical and grounded terms. They navigate the shadows and nuances of the personality while remaining highly functioning in their careers and relationships. Regardless of past experience or beliefs, one can be surprisingly accepting or terribly thrown off by a life-threatening illness. Conversations about death are most generative when we listen for our inner wisdom as well as for that of others. Remaining open and flexible is helpful, and sometimes giving silence its due is essential.

A frequent barrier to generative conversation is a misalignment of position or awareness between the parties speaking. One person might be speaking very rationally about the merits and weaknesses of a particular treatment while the other might be talking emotionally about what feels safe or reassuring. One might be talking about what is good for the individual while the other is focused on the entire family. One might be pondering immediate concerns while the other is contemplating the future. The conversation becomes even more complex when the individuals involved are at different stages of development. Just as there are stages of physical and cognitive development, there are also levels of emotional and spiritual development. Sometimes it seems like someone is being very stubborn when the truth is they simply do not have the requisite learning to understand the other's position. This can be misinterpreted in

GENERATIVE CONVERSATION

countless ways and often ends with an agreement to disagree or worse. If we want the relationship to remain intact, we need to keep trying to learn what is informing the other person's point of view. If they simply have not had the kinds of experiences that would help them to see a certain point of view, they cannot be blamed for failing to understand. In a generative conversation it is not important to be right or to win the discussion. It is more important to nurture the relationship until time and experience can do their work.

We all want to be understood, and the need can become more urgent if we feel we are running out of time. However, many people are not understood until long after their deaths. Ideas that seemed radical and impossible turn out to be shockingly accurate and useful. Art that was too avant-garde and dissonant becomes mainstream and commercial. Conversely, achievements that were highly rewarded and praised during life may quickly outlive their usefulness and be forgotten posthumously. Part of the unknown about death is not only whether or not we continue in some form beyond the body but in how our legacy ripples out through the reality we are leaving behind. In truth, this might cause us even more discomfort than the unknowable outcome of losing our body. Here again, in our hasty desire to be comfortable, we might not give the needed conversation a space in which to happen. Just as we have to allow feelings their full time and space, we have to give wonder about the unknowable its moment and place.

Perhaps the most generative conversation is like good music. Regardless of the particular concept being discussed, it has rhythm, harmony, creative tension, variation, and style. It allows for different voices and ranges, has enough structure to create meaning, and has enough improvisation to delight. It can cycle through a number of movements without losing the motif of love or the curiosity that ignites it in the first place.

THIS DAY WON'T COME AGAIN

In contemporary music we combine increasingly dissonant elements and learn to hear them as more consonant in relation to one another. We juxtapose disparate styles in ways that help us to hear them as less foreign. In just these ways, through generative conversation, we can learn to understand one another when we come from what seem like opposing points of view. This level of understanding can be especially important when we are trying to reconcile our relationships and put our affairs in order.

Some conversation, like some music, is just a ditty. It is a placeholder for simplicity in a complex world. Such conversation is comforting precisely because it is not demanding of depth or creativity. It is as familiar as a favorite pair of jeans and as soft as an old blanket. Sometimes it is like an old house when the children have moved away: quiet, but not empty. It is full of love and crowded with memories. Just because there is less to be said does not mean our togetherness is not enjoyable. When we are unwell and in the midst of the healing process, there can be a lot of this kind of togetherness. We can have an unreasonable need for every conversation to be wonderful or special as we approach death. Often it is nothing of the sort. It can be mundane, humorless, or even downright cranky. To be generative does not mean to be relentlessly innovative. It means to be life-giving. Just as time itself does not change when we are falling, life itself does not change so very much when we are dying.

The larger conversation about cancer is a different matter altogether, and keeping it generative rather than competitive is not easy. People have grown impatient that after so much expense of time and resources there remains no cure. Conspiracy theories about the suppression of cures abound, and the perceived greed of large pharmaceutical companies fuels these fires. On the other side of the conversation, a lack of empirical study and rational evidence causes frustration. For those of us

GENERATIVE CONVERSATION

whose lives have been saved by a certain approach, the conversation is often passionate. In progressive research and treatment we are starting to see an integration of paradigms that gives us much hope. With so many different kinds of cancer it is not reasonable to think there will be one universal cure. Even within an individual strain of cancer there is no one-size-fits-all. There is constant adaptation to the individual patient. With more open-source sharing of ideas and research, we can shift the conversation away from companies profiting and toward a discussion about how our species can thrive.

New treatments are making it possible to live with cancer as a chronic condition, which means we need new conversations about what that means for the quality and nature of life. Living *with* cancer instead of *after* cancer is becoming more common, and patients and caregivers need a new kind of support. A chronic condition shifts the game from one of urgency to one of endurance. Rather than abrupt changes, there are slow erosions and unforeseeable demands. We have these issues because we are alive, but the good-news part of this does not negate the grit required to grow through them and live vibrantly. Diseases other than cancer that used to result in death are now treatable, enabling people to live well into old age. Hopefully those of us with cancer can learn from having generative conversations with people who have other chronic diseases.

Whatever stage we are in, the conversations around cancer ask for courage, integrity, and tenderness. We come back to them again and again as conditions shift, and they remain generative if we are able to remain curious. They will stretch us, and, to the degree we show up, we will be rewarded with learning. Sometimes the learning will be disruptive and will result in necessary losses. At other times we may persevere and take long-standing relationships to the next level, as my dear friend and I did. No matter the outcome, if we engage with open minds and hearts, we will have an enriched capacity for living and loving. We will be more understanding of our own relationship with the inevitability of dying. We will have greater intimacy and more freedom to explore the rest of our lives. We may flourish in unexpected ways and discover new gifts to share with others.

WORK

One of the heroes I met at the cancer clinic was a man in his early forties. They had surgically removed from his abdomen everything a person might possibly live without, and he was now in chemotherapy on the same days as me. He drove himself from a town more than a few miles away and worked full-time at outdoor construction when he was not at the hospital. It was winter and I asked how he could possibly do this. He said he had used up all his sick days recovering from the surgery and he had a family to support. Another of my heroes was a woman in her seventies who cleans houses between treatments to support herself and her even less healthy, older husband. A week before she died, a different friend's husband told me he caught her down on her hands and knees washing the floor. She did not have to do that, but she wanted to.

As a self-employed person with no benefits, I needed to work through treatment too, but my gig is a whole lot easier. I work in my home studio, so I can adjust my schedule and rest between students. On days when I think I cannot possibly do it, I think of the amazing men and women I have met at the clinic and will myself to try the first lesson. I always feel better after working, and before I know it, I have made it through another day. Before my parents died, I made a video in which

THIS DAY WON'T COME AGAIN

I asked them to answer some questions I thought would be of interest to future generations. One was, "What would you like your grandchildren and great-grandchildren to know?" Mama immediately answered, "I hope they will know the joy of work."

Living with cancer changes the way we experience everything, but it does not pay the bills, remove the desire for self-sufficiency, or destroy creative passion. There are people who are too sick and disabled from treatment to hold a job, but for those of us who are able, it is a great source of strength and a part of our healing story. Because of the new ways I was learning to perceive energy and our humanity within the web of life, teaching became even more exciting and powerful. I heard my students' voices in more refined and expansive ways. Songs had more layers of meaning and beauty, my passion for supporting people to realize their expressive genius was the greatest it has ever been, and the collapse of time gave me a new sense of spaciousness and possibility. Each voice would open and strengthen in its own way, and it would move us to tears or chills when it did. My students said our transformational voice class was like going to church.

Discovering something beautiful about one's life in the midst of tragedy is why people make seemingly outrageous statements like "Cancer is the gift for people who have everything else." Facing one's mortality is a life-and-death opportunity to put everything in perspective and to stop sweating the small stuff. It is a chance to risk acting from our true nobility rather than into what we assume is expected. It is the liberty to tune into that inner guidance and actually start following it. The way this shift influences work is revelatory. Cleaning is not merely removing a layer of dirt or restoring a shine. It is touching everything with our life force. It is a chance to be grateful for the material world and to bless its bounty in our lives. Building is not just putting up another house. It is creating a home where a

WORK

family will grow and dream. Helping someone have their voice is not just for singing songs. It is for bringing truth and beauty to a world aching for heart and meaning.

In the world of cancer there are no unimportant jobs and fewer meaningless tasks. A room cleaned and free of germs can be as essential to survival as a drug accurately prescribed. A phone call properly answered can be as critical as surgery. A silent touch can do as much to heal a heart as an hour of therapy. Years of education and practice are required for the expertise and creative decision-making demanded by some jobs, while others require little or no training and are largely repetitious. Different jobs receive different paychecks, but all of the people doing them are important to the healing process and are respected and valued. This is true not only in the treatment of cancer but in the whole of life.

Some of us will not be able to continue to work through treatment. Our illness makes it impossible. This does not mean we are not working to contribute to life in other ways. My heroes at the clinic were always showing up in their greatest capacity. Although some of them were so weak they needed a wheelchair to get from the car to the building, they put on their makeup and a bright scarf. They had a big smile for everyone and remembered more names than I did. They lavished their care on the day, knowing it made a difference. We might not be able to beat cancer, but cancer does not have to beat us. Flat on our backs and pumped full of drugs, we still have a capacity to be whole in spirit and great in heart.

Cancer is not the first illness to dramatically change my life. Thyroid disease caused considerable vocal difficulty and was the reason I started teaching. I had always refused to teach, but it did not take long for me to realize that, while singing had been the career I wanted, teaching was my calling. It would never again be enough for me to have my own voice—I wanted everyone else to have theirs as well. Having cancer makes me realize it is not enough to have my own life. I want everyone to have a full life, face to the wind. As we grow into the strengths cancer calls us to, our creative force wants to share our new depths with the world as much as we ever wanted to share any expertise or abundance. The difference is that we do not concern ourselves with what we will get in return for it. We do not turn it into a job, but it is our work.

When I started teaching, I said I would always say yes when asked to sing, and I mostly give it away for free now. I am happy to serenade on behalf of the host at any party I attend. Some of my most beautiful memories of singing are times I simply gave it away because I was in the right place at the right time. Once was on an island in Greece. It was the ninetieth birthday of a prominent woman in the community, and she loved opera. When her family and friends learned that I sang opera, they asked if I would sing at her party. They said her favorite opera was *Don Giovanni*. When the time came, I stood on an overturned five-gallon pail in the piazza and sang "Mi tradi quell'alma ingrata" a cappella. Shutters flew open all around the ancient square and people hung out the windows to hear me. I felt I was in the middle of an opera as never before and the ovation was incredibly generous. It was not a job, but it was an expression of my chosen purpose to one way or another bring singing to life. I met many lovely people that evening and had an adventure I cannot otherwise imagine. Every week at the clinic I also meet someone new and lovely, and every one of them is part of my adventure of healing.

Another time I was in a small fishing village in Mexico. They were having a big party in the mango grove to celebrate the first person from their small town to graduate college. She was a beautiful young woman who had moved to the city and earned a business degree. There was a wonderful mariachi band with thrilling tenor singers. My friend asked if I would sing; she said it would be an inspiration for all the girls because the mariachi were all men and the townspeople had never heard a woman sing like I do. My precious reward was a lineup of girls who wanted to meet and hug me. My last day of chemotherapy I sang for the staff and patients at the clinic. While I was hoping to make a gift of my singing, as usual I received more than I gave when they applauded, hugged me, and wished me health.

Interestingly, I met more famous people and did more impressive gigs once I started giving my singing away. I often donate my singing to fundraisers, and some of them have been big, name-dropping events. But the big names were not the reason for anyone to be there. When I was suffering vocal breakdown from thyroid disease, I had an experience from which I began to understand a deeper purpose for being. I had to cancel an audition tour but decided to dress up in a suit and hat I had bought for it. While I was out for a walk, an elderly man approached me and said he hoped I would not misunderstand, but it was so rare anymore to see a lady so nicely dressed, he just wanted to pay me a compliment. He said it made his day. I was on vocal rest and not supposed to speak so I took out my magic slate and thanked him. I decided the message of that day was no matter what my life seemed to have come to, if I would just get out of bed and do what was left to me, it could have meaning for myself and others. It was a great lesson to bring to cancer. I do not have to be getting paid to have value. I do not have to have prescribed work to make a difference in someone else's life.

People with cancer often participate in experimental treatment. Even if it does not help them, they hope whatever is learned from the research will benefit others in the future. Just as I learned I did not have to be the one singing in order to be happy—I could be just as full when my students or friends were singing—we all seem to learn that we do not have to be

THIS DAY WON'T COME AGAIN

the ones who live longer. We just want our living to have made a difference. I think this is because we start to be aware of our place in the web of creation. We feel the energy move through us and into the world, and our sense of what is important shifts.

One of the first experiences I had of this truth was on a street in New York City. I saw an elderly woman on a stretcher being loaded into an ambulance. Her husband was holding her hand and walking beside her. My heart broke as I felt the immensity of his sadness. I said one of those quick prayers you do not even know you are saying: "God help them." At that moment a huge surge of energy went through my body and across the street to where they were. It helped me to understand something I had seen at my cousin's funeral years earlier. He died young from a motorcycle accident. At the funeral, I saw the pastor's radiance as he was speaking. It was a pure cocoon of light that moved from him and surrounded my uncle. At the moment it reached my uncle, tears ran down his face. At the reception when my uncle was thanking me for singing, he said he did not know why, but at one point when the pastor was speaking he suddenly knew his son was okay and he had perfect peace about his death. The pastor's job was to officiate the funeral, but the spirit of his radiance did the work of healing my uncle.

While getting ready for my day I was listening to the radio. It was an interview with a woman who had been pushed out of her affordable apartment by a development project, and she had been moved to a hotel for homeless people. She was raising her children in a single room there but still had a job working for the Girl Scouts organization. She saw the need around her at the homeless shelter and decided to start a new troop for homeless girls. It is Troop 6000. She was able to take the girls out of the city to a farm, and during the radio interview she shared the wonderful lessons of leadership and collaboration that had come from that adventure. While she was disappointed that her own children had not yet been moved to better and more permanent housing, she felt perhaps she was where she was needed and there were more children she could help at this homeless shelter. She had a job, but she also had a deep sense of purpose in the unpaid work her life's misfortune had brought to her. She demonstrated the spirit of resilience and healing I encounter day in and day out with cancer patients. They take my breath away with the work they do to heal our heartbroken world. They have other dreams and commitments, but they accept that cancer is theirs to do, and they do it for all of us.

When I told my oncologist I was concerned I would not be able to earn a living and make my own way in the world, he said, "You will learn to receive." Indeed there are times when all we have to bring to a day is to accept care. The grace with which we are able to do that can be significant to others. I am always deeply touched as I watch the nurses move from patient to patient in the clinic, starting intravenous lines, administering medications, taking vital signs, and doing everything in their power to make us comfortable. They are extraordinary in their ability to adapt to each personality and to avoid carrying a dynamic from one patient to another. They have developed capacities from being caregivers that many of us will never have. For patients, the primary work of treatment is to cultivate gratitude and ask for what is needed with dignity. Not everyone is equally receptive to care or able to participate in their healing. Fear, impatience, and even anger leak through the seams cancer has ripped in their personality. It is mighty work to let go of trying to control and to accept the limitations that come with cancer.

It can be difficult to think of healing as work, but it is. It is the soul's work, and we are privileged to have the time to do it. If we were to die more suddenly, we would not receive this opportunity. In the physical dimension it is often said we are what we eat. In the realm of the soul we are more likely to

THIS DAY WON'T COME AGAIN

manifest what we think and feel based on our cognitive diet. What do we read, watch, and listen to? Does it make us feel we are at war or on a journey with cancer? The way we frame and express our thoughts will dictate the nature and quality of our experience. I read about a Japanese man who had a radical remission after medical treatment had failed and he was sent home to die. He said he loved his cancer because it was part of him. He believed he loved himself back to health. That does not mean loving one's cancer is a universal cure. It means his cure was achieved in a state of love. Others are cured in a state of war. There is not a formula but rather a need at the level of the soul. The Japanese man had a fierce entrepreneurial life and needed peace and love. Another person might have always been quietly accepting and now need to stand with might. Still another might have been caught in routine and need to create a sense of movement and freedom. Someone else who always craved excitement might need routine. We each must follow our internal compass, and the unpredictability of cancer gives us permission to rely on personal intuition as never before. Once we experience giving in to our own internal guidance, it can be hard, if not impossible, to go back to living any other way.

Work and purpose may be tightly bound but are not necessarily interchangeable or interdependent. One might be retired from gainful employment, have finished raising a family, and still have a profound sense of purpose. A human life does not include a day without meaning. However, when we are flat on our backs accepting care from every direction, it is easy to question the merit of all we are going through and taking from life. Would these resources be better spent on someone else? There is too much that is unknowable for us ever to answer that question. The kindness we show a weary caregiver might make the rest of their shift a little lighter. The courage we have in the face of a dire diagnosis might inspire someone who has been paralyzed with fear. Keeping our sense of humor might make us a magnet for friendship. Our character always has a reason to be, and we never know what might evolve or when it might be needed.

Like the principle of cause and effect, a sense of purpose also can unfold over generations. We need to allow for the unknown in both the past and the future. We might not feel we have very compelling reasons for being, but our presence might be powerful for others and we will not always be cognizant of those influences. Purpose exists not only at the level of the personality but also at the level of the soul. In poetry a single word can be pivotal and shed meaning on an entire stanza. In life a single breath can be as potent as that poetic word. A purpose might not be clear today, but perhaps next week we will rise again and know our worth. I have always wondered what makes us breathe. I believe that as long as that force, whatever it is, causes us to be, our life is wanted.

For those of us who are able to stay in our jobs, it can be difficult to maintain boundaries around our new and very intense personal experience. A life-threatening illness can vastly change our sense of what is important, and we might be tempted to share our hard-won awareness in circumstances that are not designed to accommodate such conversations. We might be working as though there is no tomorrow while others feel there is all the time in the world. Even when our insights are relevant to the task at hand, if they are delivered with undue urgency or without permission, they are not likely to have a positive impact. Sometimes it is necessary to talk to coworkers and employers about what is changing for us so they can understand and support us, but we have to remember we do not get to change everyone else to suit the phase we are in. We might have to move to a new job that is a better fit for our burgeoning awareness. This level of upheaval when we are in treatment can seem as overwhelming as losing key personal relationships, and yet trying to sustain the status quo can be impossible for everyone involved. Sometimes a gift of cancer is to move us into a new career that is more fulfilling because it demands more and we now have the awareness and experience to meet those demands. Cancer does not necessarily diminish our capacity for work. It just might expand it. We cannot easily compartmentalize the life force it takes to heal.

Some of us will have stronger rather than weaker boundaries. We might find ourselves in a workplace where there is gossip or a lot of unrelated activity with people who are not dedicated to their jobs. We might be less inclined to participate or even tolerate such behavior because our brush with mortality makes us value our time too much to give it to negativity of any kind. If we have not always been so clear about our preferences, it can be very difficult to change our behavior without making waves. Certainly this reality can be an issue whether we have cancer or not, but sometimes illness brings us to the tipping point where we have to confront it. These are the aspects of work that fatigue us to the bone when we are already being pushed to our limits by so many other factors. All of these issues with work are even more complicated when the benefits we need to cover our treatment depend on our staying put in a job or career. This is another place where professional support can be a godsend. A very popular cancer support group in my community deals solely with navigating the return to work.

Another interesting shift is that we might spend less time working but get just as much if not more done. Because cancer has a way of stripping away the nonessential, there is an ability to focus intently on a particular matter, to achieve better results in less time. Because we fatigue more quickly, there are periods of rest that can be surprisingly full of revelation and inspiration. Such creativity does not always arise when we simply plug away

WORK

at a project. This rhythm of effort and release is being explored in workplaces where everyone is perfectly healthy and it is yielding some positive results. It is another one of the surprising gifts of cancer when we do not resist it. Of course, a trap is to fall into laziness and use illness as an excuse to be less productive, but most of us who face death and cherish life are unlikely to be satisfied to fritter away our time, especially at the expense of others.

Work might also become more playful with the perspective cancer gives us. While some of us certainly become more serious about the things we want to accomplish, many of us feel that if we are ever going to have fun we had best get started. We get just as much if not more done in a lighthearted way. We have time for a kind word when a colleague is struggling. We enjoy a little teasing and a bad pun or two. We might find this playfulness actually improves our creativity, and our work takes on a shimmer of excellence that was not there before.

I remember reading somewhere a bit of advice that said, if you are wondering if your work is done, ask if you are still here. Sometimes cancer stretches us beyond capacity, and the only work that remains is to let go of all expectation. Our job is to take nurture for all dimensions of the self and to rest. Whatever stage of productivity we find ourselves in, the work of daily living goes on. Needs and wants shift with time and circumstance and they are different for each of us. Because of that uniqueness, each and every breath is ours to use as only we can. It is wanted. We are wanted. Our opportunity is to create heart and meaning for ourselves and to spend it to support others. This is the work of love, and it is never done.

GOING FOR THE GOLD

Olympic athletes train a lifetime and risk everything to go for the gold. What they do is thrilling. It is no wonder we watch and celebrate them. They remind us of our human capacity for greatness. I know we all cannot be gold-medal Olympians, but we all can live up to our highest potential. I sometimes wonder if, because our culture gives so much power to wealth and fame, we forget other elements of our greatness, and we fail to include how expansive and capable we become through our connectedness with one another, with nature, and with spirit.

When athletes stand on a podium, those coveted gold medals they receive belong, in part, to every child who raced against them from the time they learned to run. They belong to every school and college athlete they ever competed against. They belong to every trainer and researcher who has contributed to the evolution of their sport. They belong to the designers of the gear they wear and the workers who manufacture it. They belong to the architects and builders of the facilities in which they have competed. They belong to the farmers and producers who have fed their table since birth. They belong to everyone who prayed and cheered. No one wins a gold medal without the contribution of countless people connected in ways we may take for granted or even be unaware of.

GOING FOR THE GOLD

Every time someone survives cancer as a result of the treatment they receive, part of their recovery story includes all those patients who participated in an experimental study, with all the researchers and caregivers who have worked in cancer clinics for generations. Every success story includes many who tried and died. Their dreams live in today's survivors. A cancer diagnosis that has a poor prognosis could make it seem like the best days of life are suddenly and heartbreakingly over. In my experience, nothing could be further from the truth. No matter where I am in the progress of disease and healing, every day delivers some measure of revelation and wonder. Every day is an opportunity to witness the greatness of the human spirit and to celebrate the significance of someone's story, however anonymous or unsung their lives might be.

Personal recovery from cancer occurs as the result of many small, unremarkable actions, and it can feel like you will never be well again. As soon as possible after surgery I was up and walking the hallways of the hospital with my medication tree. In a couple of days I was home and climbing the stairs to my second-floor apartment. Every day I took a walk, though it was harder without the painkillers. Little by little, over a period of months I was back to walking my usual distance, though not at my old pace. It was still hard to imagine I would ever be as fit as I was before I became ill. Then one day my feet just moved faster, my arms swung higher, and I power walked almost the entire distance. Every slow and painful step had moved me toward my goal of recovering physical fitness. Global cures also come about as countless patients, caregivers, and researchers take the small steps that work together to generate unprecedented solutions. Our challenge is to be prepared to take those steps when we are in the right place at the right time. We prepare by doing what Olympic athletes do: we practice.

If we want to become the grace we are capable of being in the world, even with cancer, we can begin a practice of going for gold, of living into our greatness by meeting the given challenge in any moment. We cannot always say we will recover from cancer or regain our complete vitality. However, we can take the ordinary actions that build stamina and lead to resourcefulness. We can start a journey toward excellence at any time, and we have no idea where those first painful steps might take us.

I had a wildly passionate desire to sing. I thought I would rather die than live as anything but a singer. Then illness came and my world expanded. Suddenly there were thousands of things to live for. There were details in every moment I could not possibly attend to before another moment lavished itself upon me. There were gifts of perception and revelations I had not imagined. I did not regret the life I had lived pursuing my dream of performing because I would not wish away the riches and lessons I had achieved, the love I had experienced, or the person I had become. I simply realized that part of my life was over. Something else was calling to me, and I knew I was going to follow it. This is happening again with cancer. I am a changed person with a new direction.

The spirit of creative direction often speaks to us through dreaming or vision, but we can find it hard to follow when we are not sure if it is a true vision or just a fantasy. Fantasy is a pleasant diversion in which we do not imagine the amount of practice it might take to achieve our dream—we go straight to the acceptance speech. Then we carry on with our lives and do not take a single step toward making our fantasy a reality. Vision, on the other hand, can feel too big to achieve. It is hard to know where to begin, but it will not let go of us. It feels like we will have to risk everything we have and everything we are in order to manifest it. This is where the advice to keep our eyes on the big things so the little things go in the right direction comes in handy. We envision what we want to manifest and then we come down to earth and decide on this day's tasks. We keep our eye on the cure, and then we participate in the treatments or research trials that are available to us today.

One of the most mystifying aspects of true and deeply rooted vision is that circumstances often conspire to help us achieve it. We are wowed by the synchronicity that accompanies it. I was invited to an Indigenous full-moon circle in New York City. As the talking stick was passed around the circle, a woman named Barbara spoke of needing help to take her art into the world. I knew some gallery owners, so I gave her my business card. When we met for lunch she told me about her practice of going into vision and listening to Great Spirit. She told me that for years, upon entering into vision, dark forces had pursued her and tried to steal an imaginary amulet Great Spirit had asked her to protect. At one point in a vision she was so exhausted by the danger, she threw the amulet into imaginary quicksand. Great Spirit reached into the sand and placed the amulet back in her hand, saying, "I asked you to protect this for me." A few months later she was at a *naraya* (an American Indigenous dance) and a man she did not know said, "Wait here. I have something for you." He brought his wife over and gestured to Barbara, saying, "This is the woman." His wife took a pouch from around her neck and gave it to Barbara. Barbara asked what it was, and they said, "You'll see." Later, when she was alone in her room, Barbara opened the pouch and saw the amulet she had been protecting for years in her visions.

She took this gift as an omen and renewed her vow to Great Spirit. She just wanted to serve and would do anything that was asked of her. She was then given a vision of a sculpture and told to create it. "But I'm not an artist," she protested. Spirit said, "I thought you told me you would do anything for me." So off she went to take art classes and learned how to make the sculpture. It was like this with every piece of art she was shown: she had to study and learn how to realize the vision. The practice of protecting that amulet prepared Barbara to go to extremes in order to make the art she envisioned, and that artwork prepared her to be an activist on behalf of her tribe. Over the years I knew her, she was guided to lead her people through legal battles to reclaim sacred sites. One was a hot spring that had been paved over and turned into a parking lot, another a sacred rock that climbers had defaced.

Sometimes I wonder if we are asked to do things we do not think we know how to do because we are less likely to try to control the process or outcome at the level of our personality. Maybe we are more likely to follow what Barbara and many others call guidance when we lack the wherewithal to construct an alternative. It is like this when we decide on a treatment plan for our cancer. We rely on recommendations from experts as well as on gut feelings within. We make our choices knowing there are no guaranteed outcomes. It is an exceptional act of willingness and an inspiring expression of the life force.

Cancer comes to us at different stages of our lives. It came to me after a lifetime of small illnesses that had, in retrospect, actually prepared me for it, not unlike the way Barbara's life prepared her for her activism. To others cancer comes early, before there has been a chance to live dreams or learn from failures. To some it comes when they are elders. Going for the gold while healing from cancer will look very different depending on the stage of life we are in and what is calling to us at the time. There is no prescribed path, but whatever way we choose will be peopled with those whose grace is to go there with us. We all are contributing to the pinnacles of human performance, whether it is as athletes, artists, or patients. We are part of the web of humanity that both supports and evolves from individual endeavor.

When we practice seeking and listening to internal guidance, it does not always make sense or seem possible. We often do not turn within until all else has failed, until the tension and conflict have become unbearable. But the guidance we receive, rather than bringing comfort, might bring healing by pushing us beyond our perceived limitations. Instead of things getting easier, we are often led to take increasingly challenging actions. Sometimes they are to benefit ourselves, and at other times we will take them on behalf of others. Where cancer is concerned, our gain is not always health. Sometimes it is an increased capacity to love.

The creative process by definition requires us to endure the tension between the conception of an idea and its manifestation. Sometimes it is a few hours, sometimes months or years, sometimes more than a lifetime. Sometimes when we get that horrible prognosis, we go for the gold by participating in a drug trial that lists side effects that sound as awful as cancer itself. We risk the odds and find ourselves living in a way we had always admired in others but thought we would never have the strength to achieve ourselves. We know the trial might not cure us, especially if we randomly end up in the control group. Still, we dare to hope our participation will help others win the race against cancer.

While I was recovering from my first surgery, my friend Lisa shared a documentary film called *Crazy Sexy Cancer*. The filmmaker, Kris Carr, left no stone unturned in her determination to live in spite of an incurable cancer. Her fierce journey included a passionate love affair that led to marriage. How many of us would assume the possibility of marriage after such a diagnosis? But then again, who would be a more compelling partner than someone who knows how to live all the way to the edges of every day? She was an actress who went for the gold and kept her art alive by making a movie of her life with cancer. She shares everything that helped her and tries to support others as she reveals both the heartbreaking drama of cancer and the soaring ecstasy of living into her greatness in spite of it.

Guidance does not come only to special or experienced people. It comes as readily to unknown or young people like Maggie Doyne. Her book, *Between the Mountain and the Sky*, tells her story of traveling to Nepal during a gap year between high school and college. She met a young girl breaking rocks in a quarry and decided to invest the five thousand dollars she had saved to buy a parcel of land and build a children's home. She launched the BlinkNow Foundation and started a tuition-free school for more than four hundred students. "[She dreams] of a world that cares for its weak, its sick, its handicapped, its widowed, its orphaned, its vulnerable. And a world where love rules. Love of all kinds." Her work has been recognized around the world, and she has changed the lives of hundreds of people.

Terry Fox decided to run his Marathon of Hope, and, like him, many people with life-threatening and debilitating illnesses do all manner of things that release their greatness into the world. Stephen Hawking was an exceptional example of how someone fully engaged in living was able to defy all probabilities and go for gold. Inspired work and greatness do not cure diseases, but they illustrate the incredible power of healing to extend a life and fulfill its legacy. We learn from others that no matter our state of health as we live with cancer, we still have genius, and it is ours to spend.

One of the humblest paths to greatness is gratitude. I heard an amazing example of this at a performance I attended. As I recall the story the singer told that evening, he had been diagnosed with a malignant tumor in his ear. From his research on the internet he learned that people had been quite mangled by the surgery, lost their hearing and more. This was not a good option for anyone, but especially not for a musician. However, there was a new kind of surgery that was having great success

GOING FOR THE GOLD

and leaving people intact. He decided he had to have this surgery, but his insurance plan would not cover it unless he could find a doctor who would write a letter saying it was a superior and necessary treatment. None of the doctors he approached would do that. They considered it experimental and dangerous.

Finally, he found a doctor who was not even settled in his office—he was still unpacking his boxes. By this time the singer had a substantial stack of papers and evidence supporting his quest, but the doctor still said he did not believe it was the best option. However, he believed patients had a right to choose their treatment, so he wrote the letter.

After a successful surgery and complete healing, the singer thought he should write a thank-you card to the doctor who had written the letter of referral, but he kept putting it off. Finally one day he realized he could have written several thank-you cards in the time he had spent thinking about it. He sat down and did it. Sometime later he received a letter from the doctor who said he was so impressed by the results of the treatment, he went off and learned this new kind of surgery himself. He was now using it to treat his patients. The musician ended that story by saying he thinks the most important thing he has ever done—more important than winning prestigious awards or having a successful career—is to write that thank-you card. Gratitude is commonly recommended for healing ourselves and improving the quality of our lives. From this exquisite singer I learned how expressing it could move gratitude out of our own loving hearts into the world, where it can inspire change and facilitate healing for countless others.

If we cannot be thankful for cancer, perhaps we can be thankful for who we become as a result of it. We can be thankful for the developing resources and capacities we had never experienced in ourselves until now. Untapped courage and determination, resilience and humor, endurance and humility emerge as necessary. Like physical recovery, they do not arrive fully evolved. They are earned in hundreds of small choices to laugh instead of cry, to risk instead of rely on what seems safe. Perhaps blind faith is the single most important ingredient in listening to our inner impulses to just try. So often we ask how we can know the still, small voice telling us what to do is right. We cannot know; because of our faith, we do it anyway.

I remember once racing home in a downpour, but instead of heading into the nearest subway entrance I turned down a street that was not the most direct route. What, I wondered, was I doing? I would be drenched, and as a singer my overwhelming thought was that this surely would not be good for my voice. It was as though something had borrowed my feet and was having its way with me. Another block down the street I came upon a friend from out of town at a pay phone trying to call me to ask if we could meet for coffee. How many times do we override these subtle promptings and inexplicable urges?

It is tempting to think of faith as some huge thing that allowed heroes such as Mahatma Gandhi to lead India to independence. But he and so many others like him are just the ones "on the podium." Rosa Parks refusing to move to the back of the bus was pivotal to the Civil Rights Movement, but she was not the first or the only one to refuse to move. Because of the timing, she was like a match adding fire to the Civil Rights Movement. Martin Luther King Jr. decided to serve that movement with a dream that was larger than his own life, and it lives on today. It will live as many tomorrows as it takes for the dream to be fulfilled. He and Mother Teresa and Nelson Mandela and Gandhi and so many others demonstrate that ordinary people can overcome oppression and poverty. We can provide refuge and heal broken social structures. We can recover polluted ecosystems and negotiate peace in genocidal war zones. We can cure illnesses, and when we cannot, we can live wholly and unapologetically into the rest of what remains to us. We can take the small and cumulative steps that propel humanity to its next level of excellence.

We might find it hard to believe that the way we live with illness is as vital as the achievements of famous people we remember and admire, but it is. Every relationship we have during treatment, recovery, and dying is touched by the quality of our life force, by the beauty of our interpretation, by the wonder of our desire. As my friend Lori says, "Together we have the opportunity to re-enchant humanity."

Our world is a sensual paradise teeming with wonders and stitched together with miracles. We call on those miracles because this world is also a troubling place. But maybe our troubles are of the "right kind" to catalyze our capacities to heal, both personally and collectively. What troubles us calls us to our depths, where we meet our unique genius and creative capacities. We rise into our greatness and allow ourselves to be used as instruments for miracles when we make ourselves available to meet the challenges before us.

There is nothing too big or too small to do or to share, no individual more or less important to this sprawling, magnificent evolutionary story. When we devote ourselves to realizing a true vision, we can act with service, gratitude, and faith. We can work toward something not because it will be successful but because it is the right thing to do. We can take every step toward health with the prayer to be cured and the confidence we will be healed. The practice is to listen to that spirit within so that when it asks for our hands, or our feet, or our voice, we answer, "Okay. I'll do that."

CELEBRATION

There are two cymbals at the cancer-treatment clinic—one outside the chemotherapy unit and another outside the radiation unit. Several times a day the waiting rooms erupt in applause as someone strikes a cymbal to celebrate finishing treatment. We are not celebrating being cured—it is too early to know if that has been achieved. Sometimes we receive treatment not for a cure but simply to alleviate symptoms and improve the quality of our remaining days. We still may strike the gong to celebrate. Celebrating in the presence of terminal illness and the shrinking possibility of living one's dreams is poignant and important. There is gratitude for this day and the grace of what we are given. Humor has not abandoned us and there is still a capacity for joy. It abides in the heart that powers the hand to strike that cymbal.

As I write this, we have just come through the biggest holiday season of the year. It is timed around the winter solstice, and one way or another all our traditions seek to bring light to a dark time. I wonder though if in our desire for light we fail to celebrate the gifts of longer nights that invite us to stay quietly home. We may find healing in being still, sleeping longer, and dreaming in different states. It may be a time to reflect on the past growing season and to imagine what to seed in the coming

CELEBRATION

one. Instead we busy ourselves with excesses and push through exhaustion toward another season of acquisition. What does this mean to one who is eyeing the future from the perspective of a life-threatening illness like cancer?

I have come to think celebration is not so much a date or a function, but rather a state of radiance. In Mexico I had the honor of meeting a priest who had been kidnapped and tortured to within an inch of his life. He might be the most radiant person I have ever personally known. He said that while he was being tortured he went into a state of bliss and felt deep compassion for the men torturing him. He prayed that they too might one day experience the ecstasy he was in.

He celebrated Christmas Eve mass with his congregation in a tiny village, but his reputation had traveled far and wide. People came from miles around to receive his blessing. Farmers brought their animals large and small to be blessed as well. It was impossible for everyone to fit inside the small church, but I was fortunate enough to stand at the back.

Parishioners inside and out sang to the lilt of guitars. The Christmas pageant was enacted with a young couple playing Mary and Joseph. When it was time for the sermon, this beloved priest held their newborn baby up to the congregation and said, "This is the Baby Jesus!" Everyone cheered. Then he held another child up and said, "And this is the Baby Jesus!" More cheering and laughter. He lifted several more children, girls and boys of various ages, and said each time, "And this is the Baby Jesus!" Each time the cheering and laughter grew. Then, in the final quiet, he said, "You are all sons and daughters of God. Love God, love each other, and live in peace." That was it. Then for several hours he stood in the churchyard and gave an individual blessing to each person and animal in line. Nothing has ever felt to me like a truer celebration of light and life.

105

THIS DAY WON'T COME AGAIN

Once you have had a revelation and ecstasy in the midst of the worst thing that could ever happen to you, there is a simplicity and clarity about life. Every day can be a celebration. This is a gift many of us attribute to cancer. This is the spirit I have felt arising in me these past few years. I say it is arising because I have not mastered living into it, but I do recognize it. It is an uncomplicated reverence, a quiet urge to smooth the creases in a rough day with gratitude that every moment is a potential threshold to ecstasy.

Celebration is, first of all, an observance. There is often a specific location and ritual that accompanies observance as celebration. The clinic became one of those locations for me, and earlier I referred to it as a temple. I always tried to dress festively and put on my makeup for treatments. I said I was preparing for my miracle. There was the weekly ritual of checking in, going for blood work, getting the okay from the oncologist, and finally the intravenous medication. Then came the hours of resting and receiving, of lucid dreaming and the collapse of time. How better to observe and celebrate treatment than to drop into one of those deep states of concentration where we slip through the structures of time?

Celebration is also the act of praising. I wonder if there could be any greater praising of life than to try, at any cost, to save it. The conversation most of us had at the clinic was one of gratitude for a little more time, for a reason to hope there would be enough tomorrows to live just one more dream into reality. Praise for research, praise for caregivers, and, yes, praise for God. There was praise for the nature of the day, its brilliance or calm, its blossoming or freezing. The pure pleasure of sensuality became a celebration of the unlikeliest of details. How better to praise than to be lost in wonder at the unexpected revelation of a moment, an occasion, a becoming in which we cannot contain the radiance bursting through the seams of our knowing?

CELEBRATION

And celebration is to proclaim. Unlike praising, which is a festival of appreciation that can brighten any moment, proclamation is calling us to witness a truth that calls for celebration. We are a day or a year older. We have been married fifty golden years. A child is born. A beloved dies. These are measures of time as sure as sunrise. We adorn them and attend them. How better to proclaim than with an unscripted presence, an innocent willingness, a playful spirit that does not need a thing but its flesh-and-blood creativity to make a party? At a gathering in honor of his moving for new work, the priest I mentioned found a way to speak to everyone: he took a large black garbage bag, went to each person, and collected all the paper plates. While doing so he thanked everyone for their presence at the party and in his life. In the role of a servant he celebrated the years he had been with them.

The celebrations that come with cancer are full of significance and surprise. We celebrate a successful surgery, the end of invasive treatment, and especially news of a promising prognosis. We celebrate being able to keep a meal down or being able to carry our own groceries up the stairs—anything that says our strength is returning. We celebrate acceptance into a research trial when everything else has failed. We celebrate living past the weeks or months projected. We celebrate the end of suffering. In the midst of all of this we celebrate anniversaries and achievements we dared to dream we would live for. We celebrate the lives of those who die before us. There is a bitter sweetness to every one of these occasions—the delight that we are here for it and the poignant possibility we might not be next year.

Sometimes when people are diagnosed they say they wish they had been suddenly killed in an accident. They would rather not know death is coming. Dealing with goodbyes and putting their affairs in order brings nothing but distress. They want no part of it, and they are certainly not up for a celebration.

THIS DAY WON'T COME AGAIN

Fortunately, there are people who celebrate us in spite of ourselves. We do not have to be chipper or in good humor to celebrate. Celebration can be the very thing that puts us in a happier mood, and thankfully gentle individuals convince us to participate. One of the reasons we do not have rules that govern behavior at the end of life is because it is impossible to know what will be important or needed by each person. That includes the needs of loved ones as well as those who are ill.

Sometimes people show up for us. Sometimes, in spite of our diminishing health and the knowledge that our time may be limited, they do not. People have their own lives and obligations that do not change because we are having the best or worst of times. Expectation and attachment are no better friends during illness than they are in good health. People will be with us and for us when they can be. They will disappoint us knowingly or unknowingly. These are aspects of relationship that are always at play around our desire or need to celebrate regardless of the state of our health. Like everything else, celebration has a shadow, and cancer has a way of shedding light on it.

I take a page from the age-old story of the wealthy man who threw a banquet for his friends. They all made excuses for why they could not come, so he invited the poor and needy to take their place at his table. I am reminded that celebration is not dependent on specific people. It is our state of being that creates the experience. If we are radiant with the celebration of our life this day, we will be a light. Someone might see that light and join us.

Some people think it is disrespectful to celebrate or be happy when someone is nearing the end of life. This is true if patients need quiet and stillness for any reason, and especially if they are dealing with great physical discomfort. But this is not the circumstance for everyone. As with so many other things in life, if celebration is part of wholeness and loving, it is as much so at the end of life as at the beginning.

CELEBRATION

We have even taken to calling a funeral a celebration of life. We focus on the grace of the person who has died, observing, praising, and proclaiming their achievements and qualities. We also use this time to create meaning out of the suffering and challenge of a life. We celebrate humility, tenacity, and faith. We praise the qualities that enable someone to redeem a life from the tragedy of oppression to the triumph it wins for future generations. It is a time to celebrate the love that grows in the hearts of those still alive. But no matter how we embrace the radiance of a life well lived, there is loss and grieving. Even as every celebration is the beginning of something new, it is also the end of what has been. Even when change is wonderful, it asks for new depths, and our experience of it depends on what we bring to it. Death asks so much more from us because it is so final.

Celebration requires imagination and creativity in order to have meaning. It may be prompted by culture and tradition or called by circumstance and need. The most important thing is that it be fulfilling. For some of us, one of the great gifts of cancer is that often it gives us time near the end to put our affairs in order. There is time to think of our legacy, to settle unfinished business, and to create meaning from our lives. One friend had only five weeks between diagnosis and death, but in that time she was able to interact with everyone who had been important to her. I was deeply touched and grateful she included me.

Sorting through our belongings can be one way to celebrate all we have lived. Things remind us of those we have loved and the important moments we shared. They help us cherish the family we raised and the lives that go on because we were able to be a vessel for them. They help us acknowledge the pivotal milestones of our education and career, the service we did for others. We think of what we took and what it meant to us to ask and receive. In every instance we consider what life has brought to us and who we have become as a result of it.

109

THIS DAY WON'T COME AGAIN

I love giving gifts, but I do not wait for rituals, anniversaries, or achievements to celebrate. If I see something in a shop that I know should belong to someone I love, I purchase it and give it to that person right away. I do love special occasions and think they are hugely important, but I am most likely to show up at them empty-handed. I tend to be more interested in the energetic than the material elements of celebration. I am more captivated by the expressions of the heart than the exchanges of merchandise. At times I think this lack of materialism has been one of my shortcomings, because it overlooks the importance of mementos and the treasures that travel with us through time.

These items have importance to us and in many ways tether us to existence. We often celebrate our love for one another by exchanging material gifts. We also acquire things to support our living and enable us to better share our grace. In times when life is uncertain, it is not uncommon to wonder if anyone might like to have our treasures to use and remember us by. I kept sweaters from my parents when they died and wore them to chemotherapy. I kept my father's flannel bathrobe and some of my mother's jewelry. I wear these things every day with deep joy and gratitude. So who in my life would like to feel me close when I leave this body? What would I share with them at the end of my days to celebrate our loving and the knowledge that love will outlive our death? What might they ask for? What really is the "stuff" of life?

These questions fuel the quiet process of sorting through endless details and accumulated treasures. Some of my loves have known exactly what they need to give and to whom before they say their final goodbye. Many have substantial possessions and properties, several children, and very difficult decisions to make. These are matters for wills and legal professionals. The items I am talking about in terms of celebrating our love are of the sentimental variety that often do not make it into wills.

CELEBRATION

I have just begun looking at this element of passage because I have acquired so little in life and feel there is not much that would be of value to anyone else. I barely have anything to mention in a will. However, I am learning that there are places for some of my possessions, and they can make a difference. I knew I would never wear certain performance gowns again. I had them dry-cleaned thinking I could possibly take them to a consignment shop. Then I saw a Facebook post asking for donations of gowns to give to girls who could not afford prom dresses. My gowns found a home that makes my heart sing. I also have some lovely artwork. A couple days ago someone came to dinner and fell in love with one unusual piece. Now I know where that belongs. Since I have started, I think two or more people might want the same thing, and I will have to disappoint everyone but the person who receives it. This choice is hard, but I am starting to know where these items belong and why. I understand the meaning and joy they have brought to me, and I know where they are being called. I recognize the lessons of attachment and disappointment are not all mine. I cannot control everything or make people happy any more at the end of days than I could at any other time in life.

Not everyone feels called to deal with their possessions, and not everyone is able even if they would like to. I have faith in each process and the people who end up doing the work. In my old apartment building the task sometimes fell to the maintenance workers. They often made a fair amount of money from selling and repurposing items. Fellow tenants occasionally claimed other bits and pieces from the garbage room before trucks carted them away. Objects seem to find their next home just as we do.

I sometimes think my years of depression and instances of feeling suicidal prepared me for the processes that accompany the end of life. They helped me to cultivate the attitude

THIS DAY WON'T COME AGAIN

of celebrating each and every day. I was deciding to live, and I knew I had a viable choice not to. This meant there was no one else to blame if I was suffering. I was signing up for everything I got. You might argue that we do not choose to be born and have no say in how people treat us in our most vulnerable and helpless years. But there is a moment when the power of that formative time recedes and we may take life into our own hands. For me, this was when I began the slow understanding of choices I could make in order to be liberated and joyous.

I could forgive the person I was conditioned to be in my early, preconscious years. I had certain DNA that predisposed me to illness and character weakness. Not everything my family taught me was expansive enough to prepare me for a world they had never known. Some schools I went to promoted only certain kinds of learning and did not always nourish my hungry spirit.

Even though there was much to forgive, I could also thank life for who I had become. I had been born with a fierce life force that was able to endure challenges. My family socialized me well enough to leave them. I could grow away from them as much as I pleased and return to them when I utterly failed. They loved me then, and amazingly they love me now. I attended some excellent schools that blew me open with possibility. They walked me through my ignorance and taught me humility. I learned from them that I valued curiosity more than what I thought I already knew.

I could show up for the life I have today, the tempting and dangerous mystery of it. I could embrace days that fit so well it is as though they were tailored for me. I could survive days that tore through me and made death look like it would be a relief. More than anything, I could love. If I could not recognize heart and meaning in something that broke through the door, I still could create a sense of value out of the experience.

CELEBRATION

I could surrender to love and learn its ways. I could tempt life to give me another chapter so I could steal more of its secrets. I could lie with wonder all the way to morning and ask it to stay or not. Whatever life wanted, love could be my response.

Perhaps we become overwhelmed by this period of time between diagnosis and the final celebration of life because of what we regret. For decades we never gave a moment's thought to all of this. We were too busy trying to get by. I do not think of avoiding, deflecting, or denying as not living—they are strategies that enable us to cope. We might wake up one day and want to try something different, but this does not mean we have to exchange choices made in the past for regret. In my experience it is better to get curious and see what we can learn. For some this might mean reflecting on the past, taking lessons from it, and making amends. For others who will not have time or inclination, it might simply mean choosing differently now. Sometimes the greatest change we can make . . . is to change.

We do not have to fret about the end of our time on earth. Just as situations created by previous generations were passed on to us to deal with, so future generations will inherit our unfinished business. No one completes everything. It is impossible to live into one's entire potential. Everyone has had to make choices, and each wonders about the roads not taken. We have the opportunity to forgive ourselves and celebrate all we are learning and becoming. We can change things now, through the nobility of how we live and die with cancer.

Some of us will leave our celebration of life to those who have known and loved us. Some deep wisdom within us senses they will create what they need in order to feel complete. Some of us will look after the details as our final expression or gift to our loved ones. It is not that any way of doing this is right. Nor is it wrong to seek someone else's way because we do not have our own. It is just another opportunity. For those of us who

THIS DAY WON'T COME AGAIN

need to do it, we may surprise ourselves with the beauty and joy of it. As with so many other things, the synchronicity can be absolutely delicious.

Mostly the decisions we make will be based on our sense of who will miss us most and what we can do to comfort them. Our choices will be our final attempts to express the love pushing against the walls of our chest and thrashing against the bondage of our humanity. More than anything, we have wanted life to somehow express the infinity of love we sense but can never hold. We cannot take or give this radiance because we all already have it. We share it with all of creation from our first to our final breath. We talk about miracles in plural, but really there is only one. It is the radiance of love. This is the stuff of life. This is what we celebrate, and need to celebrate.

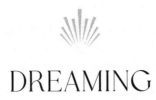

DREAMING

When my friend told me about her experience of going someplace wonderful during a surgical procedure, I realized it was more than a dream and more than real to her. It was a visit of sorts to an indescribable dimension, and she wanted to return to it. As I listened I saw how the telling of it transformed her. It had a numinous effect on her. This shifting of perspective overpowers every other concern in our lives. It is a kind of living large, and we never want to live small again.

Considering all the unexplained incidents in the world, it often seems as if we walk with one foot in the mystical, as though we live in parallel realities. I am not sure why we learn to accept only one set of possibilities and live in a linear progression governed by them, but once you are living on the doorstep of eternity, the distinction between realities seems less defined. Perhaps a brush with death makes it more inviting to live into other alternatives. At the edge of life there is a kind of living that colors outside the clean lines of formal structure. It likes to add shadows and brilliance and other dimensions. It likes to play with incongruent objects within the same landscape. We call it surreal, but because it startles us into such an awakened state, it can seem the most real of all.

THIS DAY WON'T COME AGAIN

There have been times when an unusual thing would occur, and then with time I would doubt it, thinking it must have been an illusion. I would assume it was impossible and decide it would be best if I kept it to myself. However, whether I had been dreaming it or not, I was pretty sure I had cancer and I acted on that intuition before doctors confirmed it. I also believe the medical records documenting spontaneous remissions from cancer are genuine. I think this sometimes happens whether we call it a miracle or not. I asked for a miracle and I believe I received it through treatment with Western medicine. I have no trouble with a miracle unfolding through time rather than instantaneously.

Unfortunately a sense of wonder and awe is not the only aspect of life that expands with cancer. So do the trials of pain and loss. We need a reason to endure the somewhat barbaric treatments we take when there is no guaranteed outcome. The closer one is to death, the less making money for its own sake is a reason to live. Money helps with ever so many things, but it does not make us immortal. Gaining status is just as ephemeral as wealth. There is no guarantee a legacy will stand up to the test of time. The things that motivate one to live are more likely to be the love you share with children, spouses, friends, a sense that you help others by being around. There is also the sensual pleasure of having a body to experience the glory of nature, or the genius of artistic creation, or the triumph of human invention. There is the pioneering spirit that lives to explore and learn as well as the homing instinct that loves to settle and nurture. There is work you adore, the architect's dream to build and the astronomer's ache to reach the stars.

The question of why we want to live puzzles me more when people persist in living but seem never to be happy with their decision. Every day is a complaint and nothing is good enough to cause a smile or gratitude. I am not saying anyone should be expected to be happy all the time. There are truly awful days, and there is no reason why someone with cancer should feel pressured to be upbeat and grateful all of the time. Discontent can motivate us to take healing action and is not always best ignored. We are not to dismiss our own symptoms with positive thinking when medical intervention can alleviate them. Nor do we have to be happy just because many things are going well. We still might wake on the wrong side of the bed and feel annoyed by nuisance. We are alive and that means we are allowed to be fully human. However, having a bad day or three is different from a constantly pessimistic mindset. That is like keeping the drapes closed and complaining there is not enough sunshine. It is important to acknowledge that those who suffer from clinical depression cannot help but see the darkness, and that is a second debilitating illness they have to cope with in addition to cancer. What I am talking about here is choosing a kind of living that misses the message in the moment. It is as though the kind of day it is going to be has been decided before it happens.

Upon waking I have no idea what is going to bubble up and how I will respond to it. I have a schedule, appointments, and commitments. They will have me working, socializing, receiving health care, and doing countless chores. But those are just titles for cells in a day planner. The choices presented while doing them is a constant surprise. I never know what song a student will ask to sing or what vocal breakthrough might come today. I have no idea what my podiatrist will talk about while he helps me grow toenails after the fallout of chemotherapy. I would never have imagined my friend would need to talk about her grandfather's attempted suicide. There's an invitation to a wedding in my mailbox and a birth announcement on Facebook. Other days are unscheduled and spacious as the prairies, full of endless sky, daydreams, and not much else.

THIS DAY WON'T COME AGAIN

Whenever possible, whether I am feeling well and happy or not, I try to watch the sunset. The white clouds turn first to apricot orange, deepen to hot pink, and finally glow a brilliant fuchsia. They darken to a purplish gray before surrendering to nightfall, the full moon and stars bright enough to outshine the city lights. I do not want to miss a moment's beauty. Nor do I want to miss a moment's challenge or learning. I have no idea if I will miss life when I am gone, so I try not to miss it while I am here.

Admittedly, I sometimes look at the troubled world and wonder why any of us want to live. It can seem to be such a mess it is hard to know where to put one's effort or hope. This heartbroken awareness of the human condition is not the idle complaining of one who refuses to open the curtains. It goes to the very marrow of meaning and it can make everything seem pointless. This is when we have to withdraw our focus from the future we hope to achieve and regroup in the present we already have. Life is not what happens after we are cured or when war is over. It is what we experience during the processes of healing and peacemaking.

What is important about my today will always be unanswerable before it happens, but while I have breath it is mine to discover and it is precious to me. There is freedom in being relieved of the burden of knowing, in waking each day to a complete mystery. I used to think this was impossible. How could one plan for a day, do outlines for a singing seminar, set goals and charge a fee without at least having some idea of how things would go? I was terrified to let go of my need to be successful. What if everything went clunk? I realized people would never get their time back and it would be up to each of us to create meaning out of the experience. I would have to trust the expression of the dream in each of us that brought us all together.

DREAMING

I do not have to get this book written, because we are connected energetically in the grid that binds life together. In other words, since these ideas have lived in me, they have lived in all of us, whether we are aware of that or not. I express concepts uniquely and narrate stories with my own particular style. My ideas or the way I express them may resonate with you because you have a similar story, and yet the way you would tell it would be distinctively yours. This is how our artistry adds its nuance to creation, and it matters. We enjoy creating and consuming all manner of things as sensual pleasures for the mind and body, but there is more than one way for evolution to take place. It will find a way with or without us. If I am not able to teach my students, they will find another teacher. It will not be the same, but it will be an amazing experience for them. If I am not here, everyone will continue loving. The world will turn, and the sun and the moon will keep their place in our sky.

We dream into possible tomorrows and make vows to love and serve, to raise children and steward the earth. If we cannot fulfill our promises, there could be suffering and heartache. When the bond between lives breaks we must find other ways to serve and to be of use. Life insists that we risk loving again and again and again. There will always be enough need to enable a working heart to find its place. And when the need is our own, we must be content to receive from another loving soul. Both giving and receiving are programmed into the natural cycles of life.

If all we want are the fireworks of life, we are destined to live under a dark sky, for fireworks do not shine so brightly in the light of day. If we can take the mundane with the glorious, we can have it all. Since having cancer, the hundreds of details each day calls me to are far more interesting. The constant challenge is in how to anchor them in the stunning awareness I now have of our radiance. I want to go past the details and pitfalls of our

119

THIS DAY WON'T COME AGAIN

personalities to the essence of our being. One of the surest routes is to see what is beautiful even though it is not always obvious.

I am not fond of sunless days, but when I grow still and watch I see a gloomy sky is layered with numerous gray hues and shapes of clouds. No two fluffy fragments are alike. They can absorb an entire afternoon's thoughts and carry them far to the east before they are rained down on another landscape. Just as rain may run off in weedy ditches and be lost to the growing season of precious crops, beauty may be lost to a flood of carelessness. This has been the story of so much learning I might have had. I accept that if I could have grown silent and receptive, and allowed a lesson to sink in, I would have. Thankfully, the learning comes at another time and in another way. In the same way the vibrant blue of a sunny day remains constant above the gathering and drifting gray of clouds, our personal radiance continues to shine within the antics of our living. The truer part of myself knows that as long as we are here we will have limitations and sharp edges. As we rub against each other we abrade the jutting corners and burnish one another's shine. Cancer makes me not want to avoid these gritty interactions. In fact it seems to move me toward them with unhinged efficiency.

With cancer it might seem there is nowhere to live but the edge, as though the center has fallen away. However, there will always be people around us who are grounded and centered in their lives. They may be reaching for us to return to them as much as we are calling for them to join us at the periphery. In the art of creating our lives this reaching for one another becomes a love song, a bridge, a boat to ferry across the wide and troubled waters.

Another disorienting possibility of this new mode of living is the temptation to wait for life to get back to normal, but you might as well want a pickle to return to being a cucumber. For a few months I have been hoping to feel better, thinking I will

DREAMING

get on with things when the ground settles, when the nausea is gone, when the joints no longer ache. But the side effects linger like a clueless guest. I finally woke the other day and admitted this might be my new best. In that case I have places to go and things to do. If something I choose is too much, I will try a different option, but I have no more waiting in me. Time, yes; waiting, no.

The surge of energy that comes with renewed dedication is essential. You cannot pretend you are inspired or that the stubbornness to keep going will be sufficient when your body needs you napping. Readiness turns its own corner and nudges you into the next stage. There are new conditions in your contract with life, an aftermath clause that allows you to move forward but only on different terms. It is a beautiful opportunity to have a new life, and once you start living it you do not want the old one back. It just means you have to believe enough in your offering to ask what you now need in order to share it.

One of my lovely houseplants has suffered along with me. As I went through treatment I failed to keep her trimmed and turned to the light. When I finally tended her I was not sure she would survive, so I took her outside. Finally, as fall swallowed the fire of summer and set the leaves aflame, my brave, beautiful plant sprouted waxy little leaves in the open soil. Before the temperature drops I need to find for her a different indoor spot with better light. We will find our new way together when I see how to move things around.

I have a friend who says if you want to change your life you should move the furniture. I admit I have always enjoyed the shifting around that makes me feel like I am in a new home. For a few days after the changes, I do not take my possessions for granted. I see them anew. Cancer can do this for life if we do not insist on returning to the old spaces our life occupied. Even if we cannot love the fact that nothing will ever be quite the

THIS DAY WON'T COME AGAIN

same again, we need not fear that life will no longer tingle with sensation. We still can dive headfirst into the pool of adventure. The thrill of the plunge does not abandon us just because we have been ill.

As much as a life review is another rich and jeweled gift of cancer, it takes inventory of debits as well as credits and can make for a wobbly period. It may take on epic proportions if reflection has not been an integral part of life, but still it is a portal into the art of dreaming anew. There is no rush, no need to push through this review. Whatever we are able to do in the time we have will be enough. If need be we can learn to do it in the space of a haiku instead of an epic poem. After all, an accounting of our life is for the enrichment of our becoming. It is not meant to bankrupt us. Its weight has already been carried, and a review is like an audit, a reckoning, so the burden of it can be set aside for the next part of our enterprise.

Perhaps the most important ingredient to living through cancer is the capacity to keep dreaming, and for me this has been hard. I have been a dreamer my whole life and have worked relentlessly to manifest those dreams. After my first round of treatment, I finished projects that already had been started and I managed to essentially close a chapter of my life before the cancer returned. This time I have to start new ventures from scratch and it is a heavier lift. For one thing, I do not feel as well. Each task requires an act of self-will and it is harder to gain momentum. Concentration is more readily hijacked and it is easy to simply fall asleep. Still, if I keep at it, eventually things come together. It is hard to act on a vision that requires time and resources when it is uncertain you have much of either. I have tended to fly solo all my life, so the dreams I have depend on my knowledge and experience to be realized. It is not possible to start them and turn them over to someone else to finish. I remind myself that it is not about finishing—it is about living.

DREAMING

It is understandable that dreams about creating something tangible become harder to entertain given their odds of being realized. Sadder to me is the loss of dreaming that is not about projects or adventures because it is, nonetheless, nourishing to the heart and soul. Fiction and poetry, music and art, dance and theater all arise from dreaming that does not worry about whether they will actually manifest—that element comes later. When we want to drift into the world of possibility, the evaluating mind needs to take a sabbatical. This is especially true when we dream of healing.

Many who care for us may worry we are not taking our diagnosis seriously, but we can dream about our death and how to prepare for it at the same time as we dream of living and all that remains possible. We do not have to dream about next year or the next decade. We can dream about next week and tomorrow. It is not an act of avoiding our present reality. We call our future into the present so it can inspire our creativity today. This dreaming is not planning. It is an adventure into unexplored territory of the heart and mind. Sometimes it sparkles and sometimes it terrifies. Either way it is another means of exploring alternative dimensions of our humanity. I feel as though I am not fully in my life when I cannot find my way to dreaming.

When I am able to dream I find myself being enthusiastically optimistic. My face naturally lifts in a smile and everyone says I look well. It is true. I look healthier when I dream, and the more I dream the healthier I feel. When I am able to dream I also am able to keep learning. Curiosity has always been a prime motivator for me, and I would like to think I could be learning right through my last breath. After all, it will be like no other. Why do I imagine learning is no longer necessary because I might die in a short while? We all are going to die. If learning ever mattered, it matters to the very end.

THIS DAY WON'T COME AGAIN

It has been easier for me to dream for those I love. I dream wonderful futures for the children, tender times for my own generation. I also dream of those who have died and the ways in which our love survives. I dream the social changes I have always worked for, a world that is fair and where coexistence is possible. I have always cared about the bigger picture, and that concern seems to have intensified for me. Perhaps it will recede as death moves closer. Who knows? There is no superior way to dream and no rating of content. As much as at any other time in life, when we confront our mortality we follow what has heart and meaning for us.

Sometimes I feel a deep kind of sorrow for myself. It is not because anything is lacking. Quite the contrary—it often comes upon me on the most perfect of days. A day when the breeze is the most delicious degree of cool to complement the warmth of the sun, when the path is lined with lemon-skinned flowers leaning to capture my attention with their radiant, round faces. This sadness haunts a golden day when the air rings with songs of insects, frogs, and birds, when trees are still and listening. It spills into an evening when the full moon rises over the mountains and makes silhouettes of ranges far in the distance. Perhaps this poignant sadness comes with beauty because one must leave it, and in the end one must leave it utterly on one's own. Or perhaps it is what some call a God-sized hole inside of us that no amount of goodness or beauty can fill. Perhaps some sadness is the longing for an even greater beauty and mystery like my dying friends have described. It is not that life is not enough, but because we dream we suspect it is not all there is.

There is no cure in all of life for this sadness. Only dropping into another state of awareness can touch it with healing. It is like illness. Positive thinking does not cure it. Something else must bring us to a quiet state where we slip through the cracks in reality to a dimension where we have never been ill. In that moment we are made whole and life goes on as though cancer never happened. It so often happens at the end of a very long period of treatment, when all else has failed. It happens because we let go of the struggle and drift into other states where such things can happen. This is where we receive a life better than dreams coming true because we cannot in our ego state dream these transformations into being. They are pure grace, as unearned as a child's love for us.

My last evening in New York City was heartbreaking. It was hard to leave the life I had made there and that I loved so dearly. My friend Sandy took me to dinner at my favorite restaurant. It was on the ground floor of the apartment building I lived in, and the people who worked there were like family. When we entered and waited to be seated, a little girl I had never seen before, not much more than a year old, began waving and jabbering. We were seated at the table behind her. Although my back was to her, she was very intent on getting my attention, so I finally turned and responded. She held her hands out to come to me. She was so insistent her parents reluctantly allowed her to go to a complete stranger. She hugged and hugged me, chattered and giggled and hugged some more. She stayed with me until her parents had finished their meal and were ready to leave. Once again I was being given exactly what I needed in order to know that somehow life was going to continue to be wonderful and full of love.

Cancer has no preferences or boundaries. It happens to you whether you like it or not. However, as you begin to feel well again and life resumes its normal chores and rhythms, its significance can become diminished. I remember talking with a friend about the sense of presence and heightened sensitivity that had returned with a second round of cancer. As we talked about the things we do throughout our lives to seek different states of being, things like meditation and prayer, she said she would not want to have cancer again but she would definitely like to live in that heightened state again. We can, but we have to choose it and work at it. Once we have experienced it, it is ours to create and share. It is our adventure and our refuge, our loss and our love. It separates us from the mundane and connects us with the unity of everything. It reminds us to dream a little differently.

I would never wish you cancer, but I would wish you the evolution and revelation it brings. One way or another, I dream that heightened aliveness may be yours today and always.

THE LOVER

When I was three years old, Papa bought a magnificent upright grand piano. I think the first thing I fell in love with was the swiveling stool. But then I touched those magical keys, and because of the way the music desk opened, I could see the felt-covered hammers strike the wires and set them ringing. I was utterly seduced by the miracle of sound at my fingertips. By following my own singing, I figured out how to play the melody of "Jesus Loves Me." It soon was followed by other children's hymns. When Aunt Virginia came to visit from Los Angeles, she taught me how to play chords, and song after song found its way through my clumsy little fingers. I had no idea about the mathematical order of music or the patterns that facilitated getting around the keyboard. I just loved the sound and singing, and I would do it any old way I could. I lost track of time and entered eternity where all my troubles turned into tunes. Nothing else existed. It was everything to me.

In a performance workshop I attended in my early twenties, we were to create a picture of our lives as singers. Everyone else drew themselves onstage with family and friends in the audience. They had homes they came and went from and pretty balanced-looking lives. I waited until the very last to share my picture. I had drawn and colored my version of a huge, yellow meadowlark in a pure blue sky. There was nothing else in the picture. The instructor asked who I was singing for. After too long a silence I finally said, "God." I did not have a clue what I meant by "God," but I was singing for something I could not call anything else. I was singing as though I was still three years old, because that was the only way I could bear to be alive.

To this day I think of the state I enter into when I am singing as a presence without and a spaciousness within. We try to explore it with science; we exalt it in art. We call it God and pray to it with every attitude known to humanity. We even fight about it as though someone's version of it could win. I have come to think it is not who or what God might be that matters. As far as I know that remains unanswerable. What truly matters is who we are, or who we become, when we find ourselves in the presence of that radiant and indescribable essence I call love.

It was spring when I realized I had cancer. Lingering traces of lilac, hyacinth, and peony blossoms perfumed the air. As I awaited medical appointments and eventual treatment, other emerald promises pushed through gray wintered dirt and sprawled into the tangle of summer gardens. I recovered from surgery as the musky-sweet confetti of autumn leaves carpeted that same dirt. Chemotherapy dripped into my veins and peritoneal cavity as moaning snow squalls buried the glories of the growing seasons. The earth was making another trip around the sun and I was still on board. I felt the preciousness of time left in me as I looked past my mortality to the prayer I meant to answer. At first, I had been startled by the thought I had cancer, but the lasting surprise was that I remained more concerned about the prayer that had come to me that morning than I was about dying. That request to be allowed to spend whatever love and grace I might be capable of had become my mantra, my entire reason for being. I felt like there was still time in me, and perhaps something else might be created if what I had

THE LOVER

lived thus far could be assembled into some kind of meaningful foundation for it. Perhaps I could become the eyes and hands and heart that could live the answer to that prayer into being.

Always I had intended to do well and to do good, but if I am to be honest, I had been governed by the need to succeed as a singer, and I thought I knew what that meant. I was driven to obtain better gigs and recognition, but I constantly undermined my progress with my unconventional ideas, my ignorance, and my untamed personality. The truth of me always surfaced in time to spare me any significant achievement. My ambition was sustained because I needed to prove I merited the O-1 visa that kept me in New York City, but in the end that was terminated anyway. I left with a heart full of gratitude that in my time there I learned more than a naive girl who started out in the bald prairie of southern Saskatchewan should have dared, and, according to my students and friends, I did accomplish some good.

While I tried to achieve the kind of success I thought was so important, I lived inside hand-me-downs and repurposed treasures. My family teased me that I drove around with my trunk open and I did not even have a car. I mostly was treated with kindness and dignity in the situations I experienced, but I never belonged in that world. I did not know how to take advantage of the contacts and opportunities I met. I had no idea how to navigate inside the halls of good fortune, and I sabotaged every chance I had. I realize now I do have genuine abilities, but they are not the kind that would achieve the dreams I chased. The most meaningful moments of my life have always been when I was helping someone else realize their genius. That is my superpower.

Years ago one of my yoga teachers in New York City invited me to an evening meditation with her guru from India. He was on a tour he called Samadhi for World Peace. Samadhi is a form of meditation that practices oneness with all of creation. He said we cannot create peace because it already exists. Our only hope is to increase its presence by merging with it, by becoming one with it. That truth changed my life. By the same reasoning, love also already exists, and we increase its power in the world by becoming the lover.

I wanted to live. Yes. Because I wanted to love wholly and I wanted to believe it was possible. But having a momentary revelation does not mean one gets to have a "happily ever after" life and be a good person 100 percent of the time. Life remains challenging enough to constantly tempt me away from my sincere intentions. Beyond the tiresome side effects of chronic treatment, my days include broken arms, crashed hard drives, missed deadlines, and one new heartbreak after another. It is not easy to consistently merge with love in the thick of chaos. More than once I have chided myself for uttering some noble-sounding prayer and then trying to live up to it, as though I could. I am not the source of love, the creator of love, the one who determines when, where, and how love flows. Either I surrender to it and let it have its way with me or I lose all sense of it. Somehow, with none of the innocence of childhood, I have needed to find some way to be with it as I did way back then while singing.

The initiation came in my early twenties. I had been essentially disowned by my father because, along with all my other sins, I was living out of wedlock with a man. My mother phoned and asked if I would come home for Christmas because the family had not been together for six years. I asked if my father wanted me there. Yes, she said, as long as I came alone.

A huge blizzard descended on the prairies, making it impossible to fly out of Edmonton, but the Greyhound buses were still running. I boarded one of the last buses to Saskatoon, certain I would be too late to make a connection to Moose Jaw, where someone from my family would meet me to make the seventy-mile drive to the farm. When the bus pulled into Saskatoon, a tall thin man with blond hair and blue eyes boarded the bus and said, "There is someone here going to Moose Jaw." I burst into tears as I made my way to the front of the bus. "We've been waiting for you," he said. My father and brother-in-law came to meet the bus in Moose Jaw, and I was going home.

My parents had built a new house, and I was given a room in the basement. That Christmas was the first time I could remember my family being together without incident. There was storytelling and laughter and a new generation whose darling antics took the pressure off. No one asked a thing about me or my life, I assumed for fear of upsetting my father. I now have the humility to admit I am not all that fascinating and there could be a lot of reasons why they found other things to talk about. My siblings left with their commotion of children before I was scheduled to leave. I was now sleeping alone in the basement and feeling pretty sorry for myself. It was true we had not angered one another, but I was not sure we had shared any love either. We had avoided everything that hurt, but I could not help but wonder if we had also failed to embrace everything that mattered.

I had to admit I had been so busy feeling sorry for myself I did not even try to do better at loving them. As I climbed into bed I noticed a light seemed to be coming through the window. Thinking the moon must be out I went to pull the lace curtains aside and take a look. The light split into two and moved toward me. Terrified, I jumped into bed, pulled the covers up, and tried to say the Lord's Prayer. I could not get it out correctly, and I was sure it was all over for me.

Inexplicably, I got really calm and asked the light what it wanted. It passed over my body and I felt what I now call a rush of spirit. I said, "It's time to talk to my parents, isn't it?" The light moved before me, out the door, and up the stairs to my parents' bedroom door. I was about to knock when my mother opened the door. We both screamed as we startled each other.

The light was gone and my mother asked if I was all right. She said they had heard a huge boom in the basement like a jet breaking the sound barrier, and she had just been getting dressed to come down and see if I was okay. I never heard that sound.

She and I and my father talked long into the night. I had always thought it was my father who had to change so we all could be safe and happy. As it turned out, it became clear it was my responsibility to make amends to him for all the ways I broke his heart, over and over and over again. I could not imagine taking responsibility for that until I felt the stirring of that light within me.

I was terrified of my father. He gave me singing and my connection to the most magnificent experiences of my life, but he also shattered me with the beliefs and passions that drove him. As I have been sorting through my history, I have been reminded of the struggle and heartbreak between us. That Christmas, the spirit of love that visited my lonely, broken heart awakened me to a calling I did not understand. It has taken decades of trying and a life-threatening illness to reveal itself to me.

When cancer came to call, I was finally ready to acknowledge the truth that none of what I had thought would bring me success mattered, other than it seduced me to risk madness and dive boldly into one adventure after another. I had been so terrified of failing that I persisted with the fantasy that, given enough time, I would figure it out, whatever "it" was. But that kind of time was done with me. All my striving and measuring fell away in the space of a heartbeat. I had what I had learned and who I had become. I needed to stop feeling embarrassed and ashamed of that so I could also accept the good I had done. That light had become my guiding force and the only way I thought I was capable of love. I had an opportunity now to utterly surrender to its greater calling with whatever was left to me.

I do not know much about how life works, but the one thing I can say with certainty is that it is outrageous. As surely as I intuited I had cancer, I decided I was going to meet a new lover. Assuming at my age and stage of health the odds might be even worse than those of surviving cancer, I nonetheless began to prepare. A friend commented that all of my living room furniture seated only one person. I had nothing to cuddle on. The next morning there was spam in my email from a local furniture store that was having a big sale. I bought a love seat. I bought new lingerie. I created a profile on a dating site for "mature" singles.

I had no idea what to say about cancer so I said nothing. When I uploaded photographs to my profile, I included a picture of myself performing original songs I recorded to raise money for ovarian cancer research. I was midway through my second round of chemotherapy and was bald for that concert, so I had decided to wear a fascinator that matched my gown. I thought if anyone looked carefully, that picture would say enough about my cancer to begin the conversation.

Six months into my membership on the dating site it was time to renew. There had been some shallow hits, but not a single one I was interested in. I decided not to continue. I assume the site boosted my profile to encourage me to renew my subscription, because my inbox was suddenly flooded with emails from prospective matches. I laughed and ignored them. For a few days. Then curiosity got the best of me and I took the bait.

In that mess of emails was one from a man who had no interest in me because he wanted someone who lived closer to him. He wrote only to encourage me, because he liked my profile and knew from his own experience that the dating game

THIS DAY WON'T COME AGAIN

could be disheartening. I responded to thank him. We began corresponding. He finally asked about the picture. In return I learned his brother had died from glioblastoma ten years earlier, and since then he had been volunteering at a cancer clinic. I told him I could not promise I would not die anytime soon, but I felt I still had something to give to a loving relationship, and I did not want to die with that left inside of me. Eventually we met, and we now take turns driving the three and a half hours of roads that separate us. We are daring to live for one another and grow in love.

I think this all started with singing as a little girl. Every time I sing, something seems to shift and move in me. There was that time in Switzerland I had just come down from the mountain and was walking through a small village in the great valley. A square, humble church caught my eye and I climbed the steps to the front door. It automatically opened before I reached it and beckoned me to enter. A plain wooden cross rose out of the concrete floor and sunlight streaming through stained glass colored the open Bible pages. The echo of my feet spiraled up through the rafters, tilting my face heavenward, and I began singing. How many prayers had these walls held and heard?

I had not been able to sing on top of the mountain. My voice was too small and the beauty too unbearable. Up there, I merged with silence and grew thin as the air. But here, in this tiny church, I could pour myself out, and the beauty breaking inside of me found its voice in the extravagant resonance of those sacred stone walls. There was nothing to ask. All that was possible was love. It was a moment I did not want to leave, but life was outside that door and it was not finished with me. It was time to return home and say my last goodbye to my father. I had already packed and sent the boxes when the call from my family came. I had a difficult time getting there, diverted again by storms and delayed flights, but that same trustworthy rush of spirit guided me home on time.

I have freedom of choice. I was created for it. When in a moment of honesty and humility about my own limitations I accidentally say one of my clumsy prayers, there is that familiar warm surge of energy. Sometimes my body becomes so electric I think I might explode into the thirty trillion cells that for some reason have come together and agreed to be Jocelyn. The miraculous is everywhere. I look out the window, and nature stuns me. I open a book, and serendipity has found a messenger to speak exactly what I need to hear. I turn on the radio and the truth of someone's story runs like a shiver through the core of my being.

These moments keep me humble and grateful. They give me faith and hope. I can't plan them. I can't control them. Left to my own devices I'm just not that good. I worry. I procrastinate. I judge. Even now, when I know I could be out of time any day, I retain a massive repertoire of untoward behaviors that interfere with my better wishes. Thankfully, none of that matters when love comes in and takes over. When that happens, I can forgive the world and life for teaching me to forget the truth about my capacity to love. I pray my way through the day and live as close to truth as I can get. I give thanks before I surrender to sleep.

Love is like air. You receive it with every inhalation. With every exhalation you decide how to spend it. I kiss the miracle of life for giving me so many days to choose, and for sending me so much love in everyone and everything I meet. The beauty of it is almost more than I can bear.

On this day of writing I have lived almost a decade with cancer, and my neighborhood has never been more lovely. The business of the world has been temporarily shut down by a coronavirus, and new roofs and porches, paint jobs, and landscaping

THIS DAY WON'T COME AGAIN

have grown out of the crack in time it created. Thrift stores are brimming as closets and garages are cleaned. Lives have been put in order and some are even running out of projects. A global pandemic has the entire community doing what some of us have been doing since we learned we have cancer. One way or another we are thinking carefully about what makes us happy and what calls our love. We are simplifying, emptying out our lives to make ourselves one with our values. We are merging with beauty and it is gushing back at us.

In the stillness of a retreat with disease, I understood I had done little more than take life for granted. I had once been a gardener, but I traded it for living in a box in the sky. I left it to others to tend to nature with a more tangible and effective love. I now fell so in love with creation it hurt. My heart, aching for the incomprehensible mystery of it all, knew I would never sustain life in the world the way I saw others doing. I would only ever be with it in the ways that are my peculiar grace.

There have been, thankfully, many times in my life where I feel like love has taken control of my personality and body. I show up and something wonderful happens that has absolutely nothing to do with how good I am, or even with my good intentions. But I have the exquisite grace of being available for something beyond my wildest dreams. People thank me, but it is not me they should thank. It is whatever it is that borrows my body and voice. What I wanted when I confronted mortality was to live consistently in this surrender to love. I am not sure it is possible, but it is what I want.

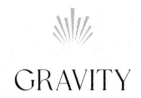

GRAVITY

I have just climbed the Niagara Escarpment to a slab bench overlooking Georgian Bay. The narrow trail has been carved by runoff rain following the path of least resistance to the Pretty River Valley. Now, in high summer at the top of the hill, the soil is dry and cracked in the pattern of a giraffe's coat. I gaze farther than I can see and get lost in the horizon, just as I did from the petroglyph hill of my childhood and the top of the Alps in Switzerland. Blue upon blue, sky and water are as still as a grass snake sunbathing in the softly breathing morning. Birds trill, insects hum, wild flowers and weeds tremble almost imperceptibly on their thin stems. We are alive!

I linger with the sensation of each breath. The air is slightly sweet and damp as the sun has not yet drawn the last of the night's humidity up into the warming sky. It is easy in this tangled patch of Eden to believe a miracle abides wherever I am, at any given moment. During chemotherapy it is more tempting to focus on better days ahead. The future, if not cancer-free, might at least be symptom-free. But the miracle actually happens when you are in treatment, not when you feel better. When you are losing your hair, your lunch, and your life as you know it is when the drugs are killing the cancer. Whether I look out on a day ravaged by human endeavor or this one ravished by nature's glory, whether I am praying for the miracle I need or cherishing the one I receive, this is a day my heart may be uplifted by hope and healing.

I do not know how much longer I will have the agility and strength to navigate the gnarly river route. They call it the Enchanted Forest and it does feel magical to me, as though everything is perfectly appointed to inspire mystical wondering. Some new hemlock trees have grown just in time to extend a branch so I can pull myself up a mucky slope. Did they know they would be needed at that precise location? Twisting tree roots and randomly wedged rocks sometimes give foothold in the steep and slippery segments along the riverbank, but in the level terrain where I am tempted to look around and daydream they trip me up. I snap out of reverie as reflexes restore my balance. Have those roots and stones been here hundreds or thousands of years, waiting patiently to call travelers present through the soles of their uncertain feet? If I had trained powers of observation and attention, I imagine I could memorize my way through these woods by their eccentric and wildly unique ways of inhabiting their territory. I could know the name and address of each tree and outcropping in relation to the directions established by the hills, the bay, and the river. I could read the guidance of the sky. But I am dull and reliant from generations of living out of our senses. Without my contemporary gadgets, I would not be able to navigate my way out of a wet paper bag.

In places the river is so tangled with fallen trees and shattered shale it is slowed to a trickle, and only by the force of gravity does it continue on to the great Lake Huron at the foot of the escarpment. Gravity exerts its force on my body too. It ages and patterns my skin like the parched dirt. It calls me to the gateway between now and next. Whether it is to nothing or everything is impossible for me to say, but gravity is law, and flow toward that passage I must. The physical body may

GRAVITY

diminish to a trickle of its youthful vitality because the force of gravity is relentless. Radiance, however, is not governed by the same laws. I learned this from my practice of yoga. I used to do a fairly rigorous practice that developed a lot of strength and flexibility. It felt wonderful to live inside that body. My practice now is to use my breath and imagination to direct my physical energy in the direction of those poses and movements. Relatively speaking, this gentler practice gives me as much nurture and renewal as the more rigorous version used to. Yoga is not only the poses; it is a practice that allows me to experience radiance within my physical body.

Radiance, the stuff of stars and creative genius, permeates the material world but is not limited by it. It enters time but can never be contained by it. We experience it when we are utterly lost in joy or elation, or anytime we transcend ordinary perceptions and break through to extraordinary revelations. It magnifies beauty and truth and ignites the fires of possibility. It illuminates unforgettable occasions, and it changes our lives forever. I think I miss a lot of miracles because my attention has been hijacked, but when I do notice them, I think radiance has burst through my limitations and rearranged the flow of my life force.

Light obeys the laws of reflection. As it dances its way through the canopy in flittering patterns between shifting shadows, it draws me into my own reflections. What I see and how I interpret it are constantly changing and rearranging me. Gazing out across the vast forest I see a stunning array of green hues carpeting the hills and nuzzling the sky. Lining the small circle of grass at the summit where I sit, individual trees are knotted and curiously shaped by years of competing for their measure of air and earth. Some have blossomed and now are bearing wild fruit. As the year rounds, the seasons strip their limbs of flower, fruit, and foliage to litter the inconstant earth. Nurture in the physical world returns from whence it came. Dust to dust.

THIS DAY WON'T COME AGAIN

The climb has worked my heart. Life also is working it, albeit in different ways. A third of one country is underwater while others are even more in drought. Almost daily there seems to be an unprecedented weather crisis in some new location. There are equal incidences of political, economic, and social instability to accompany a global pandemic. The world is starving and we need a miracle. I wanted never to lose the radiant gratitude that came with living beyond cancer, but it is harder to attain and difficult to sustain as the demands of daily living, both individual and collective, encroach on the miracle of being alive. While I rest to regain regular breathing and a steady heart, I reflect on the need to practice radiance as much as I perform physical exercise or rehearse music. Everything weakens when it is neglected. I return my gaze toward the horizon, as I have for as long as I can remember, where vision is capable of both earth and sky. I remind myself not to go back to sleep. I must protect and nurture my vision the way my friend Barbara protected the amulet Great Spirit entrusted to her. I must not grow tired and lose it in the quicksand of despair. I must allow what I am learning to rearrange both my radiant and my physical worlds.

I recall the day I left our family farm and headed for the city. I felt like I had been holding a bunch of uninflated balloons in my chest and they were suddenly blowing up and bursting free. I was speeding into the wide open prairies under that endless, living sky. I had not one clue about personal radiance, how it could light my path and shine on those I was to love. Instead, time and time again, I dislocated my power and then fought to get it back. It was messy, but I was learning that when life seemed unbearably hard, I was not alone. I was never helpless if I had anything I could give to another, and when life was amazingly good, I could shower heaven with gratitude and hope it could rain down to help another grow. I was learning, one lesson at a time, I would need to be utterly and uncompromisingly true to myself in order for life to get me where I belonged.

Cancer has brought me to a new community where I volunteer as a patient partner. There are many different projects and meetings where one can share patient experience and perspective with researchers, caregivers, and providers who seek to improve health care systems and delivery of care. I spend a lot of time listening, and often understand next to nothing, especially when a lot of acronyms are being tossed around, but even then I learn much that gives me hope. The researchers and medical staff are wholly devoted and passionate about their work. Their curiosity and tenacity peel the ordinary from the fruit of this day and show me the genius that gave me more days than I had dared to hope for. I am still alive because of a treatment they dreamed and developed, but I did not think about that or thank them for my hope and healing as my body drank the intravenous infusion.

As time passes, I cannot always determine if something I am experiencing is a side effect of chronic treatment or a product of aging. Of course it is wonderful I have lived long enough to experience aging, but I did not think it was an option, so I stopped planning for it when I signed up for treatment. Now, instead of putting my affairs in order and preparing to die, I am trying to figure out how to sustain myself as I continue living. It is the unconscious destiny of successful medical care. When choosing treatment, I was riding the momentum of my life force and did not consider the inevitable decline I will engage in until my final breath. One way or another that precious inhalation is coming to me. It is just a question of when and how.

I do not want to view aging as illness. I want it to be another stage of learning and creating, but every little twitch and irregularity could be a sign the cancer is back. I often think I should discipline my mind to forget about the cancer, but it is

THIS DAY WON'T COME AGAIN

hard to do when you take a handful of medication twice a day and endure its side effects throughout. Besides, there is something different and interesting about living with persistent uncertainty and ambiguity. Inventing a good and beautiful day in spite of its precarious nature delivers some really good opportunities.

I had an intense refresher course in my practices of living into this day during a recent hospital stay. My body can no longer tolerate the cancer medication I have taken for years. There is no cancer anywhere in my system, but my bone marrow had stopped making blood and my digestive system refused to let me eat. I lost weight and strength rapidly and had to accept that I could no longer take the medication I credited with giving me the last five and a half years of my life. I have lived longer than anyone expected, and it is not unreasonable to hope that by now the cancer will not come back. But that is not what matters.

It is tempting to give in to attachment and self-importance, to prioritize them over the commitment I made to spend the love and grace that chooses to move through me. That is not useful or life-giving. I still have all the choice and opportunity I had before this stage of illness began.

Knowing this day won't come again, how shall I spend it? That could be paralyzing when there are more choices in any given moment than anyone can ever entertain or get around to fulfilling. Furthermore, who really knows what is most important? Is it most critical to finish a creative or research project, to leave that work completed for the life that goes on without us? Is it better to spend more time with those we love, to try to embrace the coming transition and explore with one another how our love and life can go on? Or is it wisest to savor the sensual pleasures of life in a body before the world is finished with us? I suspect no choice is better than another. They are, in

GRAVITY

the end, simply different. Each brings lessons and love, and how those ripple into the future without us is impossible to know. Should we even bother thinking about what might be on the other side of this life? We can believe something all the way to the frontier of infinity, but if we are honest with ourselves, we know there is always a trace of unbelief. There has to be. It is essential for life. It is the reason we get to choose.

Despite all I have experienced and learned, despite all the delicious reflection and wonder, less has changed than I had imagined would. I live today much as I always have. There are essential chores that never go anywhere. I do them, but not always with the gratitude they merit. I partly design my time by writing tasks in the cells of a day planner, and then I throw myself at the day. I make my bed on the way out of it and take my own sweet time with the coffee I love so much. I try to keep the promises I have made. I mostly do for and with others what I said I would do. I do for myself some of what I said I would, knowing full well most things will be left undone. They are dust in the wind. They will become the soil for another lifetime. There are over eight billion people making up this day, and I bet they each have many great ideas they too will not get to. The universe is not going to run out of ideas, but you and I will run out of time.

In light of that, I wonder if the most important thing about this day might not be how to spend it, but rather who I am while I spend it. What do I truly care about? What do I still want to learn and spend in the days left to me? I keep coming back to love. Without it I cannot think of another power or quality that matters. A lot of distractions stumble into my days, and I must constantly remind myself that this world and the brief time I inhabit it may limit my life but not my love. Nothing is too big or small for love. Like the Pretty River, love has its ways of flowing through everything it encounters.

THIS DAY WON'T COME AGAIN

My eyes return one last time to the horizon. Earth and sky. Gravity and reflection. Life and radiance. My death might one day belong to cancer, but I have not lost my life to it. I gather what remains of my vim. I am going to take a different way home.

THE POETRY
OF CANCER

Written in scars
and wrinkles and stretch marks,
skin is parchment for cancer's lines
unrehearsed as birth,
indelible as death,
rhythms sprung and unlikely to rhyme,
verses open and slammed,
stories impossible to tell
without the language of love.

Written in tears
and laughter and surprise,
the face a script with cancer's edits
in the margins,
between the lines,
changes highlighted and subjects bold,
pages erased and folded,
endings impossible to know
even with the language of love.

THIS DAY WON'T COME AGAIN

Silent night bats her smoky eye,
a slit of molten gold breaks
along the shore of dreaming,
peers through life's hourglass,
still sand on both sides
of this dividing day—
the life I meant to live,
the one I never dreamed—
the day the world stood still.

Nearly perfect crime
undetected as summer's soil
beneath unbroken snow,
silent as fox,
versatile as lichen,
cancer wakes the patient miracle
biding in the temple—
light the candle,
the healer comes.

Radiance enters through the prism of time
splitting into beams of past and future,
casting unavoidable shadows
even as it illuminates
all that is inherited,
all that is dreaming,
the graceful rainbow
arcing toward healing
our numbered days.

THE POETRY OF CANCER

Living slowly as a Sunday drive,
the quiet movement of a symphony,
the blooming of a garden,
greedless senses poised
for a moment's awe,
a lifetime's consequence,
the spiral staircase
from once upon a time
to inconceivable ever after.

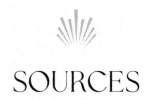

SOURCES

Page 48: "the choice might have been mistaken, the choosing was not." Stephen Sondheim, *Sunday In the Park with George*, 1984.

Page 57: "When Job's three friends . . . for they saw that his suffering was very great." Job 2: 12–13.

Page 62: "near to the brokenhearted and saves the crushed in spirit." This is a promise made in Psalm 34:18. I met a woman on a bus once who said she read the Bible to learn the promises in it. I loved that suggestion and find many beautiful promises in Psalms.

Page 63: "Two are better than one, for if they fall, one will lift up his fellow. If two lie together, they keep warm. And though a misfortune might prevail against one who is alone, two will withstand it." This is another promise, this time from Ecclesiastes 4:11.

Page 88: "While getting ready for my day I was listening to the radio. It was an interview with a woman who had been pushed out of her affordable apartment by a development project, and

THIS DAY WON'T COME AGAIN

she had been moved to a hotel for homeless people. . . . She had a job, but she also had a deep sense of purpose in the unpaid work her life's misfortune had brought to her." I heard this inspiring story on *Morning Edition*, WNYC, July 26, 2017.

Page 100: "[She dreams] of a world that cares for its weak, its sick, its handicapped, its widowed, its orphaned, its vulnerable. And a world where love rules. Love of all kinds." *Between the Mountain and the Sky* by Maggie Doyne, HarperCollins, 2022.

Page 102: "Before Rosa Parks, There Was Claudette Colvin" by Margot Adler, *Weekend Edition Sunday*, NPR, March 15, 2009.

ACKNOWLEDGMENTS

Publisher Brooke Warner, project managers Shannon Green and Addison Gallegos, and the design team at She Writes Press executed with excellence, grace, and beauty. Because they said yes, I will not die with this book inside of me.

Maria Case, artistic director of The Annex Singers, makes so many beautiful things happen in this world. She invited me to speak about hope and healing at Glebe Road United Church and then suggested the talks needed to be published. Because of her, this book was born.

Jen Hale, Maggie Hill, Sheila Kappler, and Caroline Kera were painstaking editors. Joan Ross, Heather and Don Perrier also gave careful reading and feedback. Because of them, the book became its best self.

Michelle Morgan, my wonderful publicist, for her belief and commitment. Because of her, the book will travel.

Dr. Akira Sugimoto is a brilliant and gifted surgeon and oncologist, a profound healer in every sense of the word. Because of him, I am still living into my dreams.

Heather Shaddick, a wise, compassionate, and tender soul, graciously helped me learn how to live with cancer. Because of her, I am more than a survivor.

THIS DAY WON'T COME AGAIN

I watched heroic nurses, technicians, staff, and volunteers at London Health Sciences adapt their caregiving with kindness, creativity, and humor to meet the needs of every individual patient. Because of them, treatment was bearable.

The Wellspring community offers ongoing healing and support to survivors and caregivers. Because of them, new friendships are part of the journey.

Family and friends showed up with care and kept me pointed toward hope and healing. Because of them, I have never been alone.

My students kept coming for singing lessons and thoughtfully accommodated my needs. Because of them, my life pours out in endless song.

Doug Thompson took a chance on a woman with chronic ovarian cancer. Because he loves me . . . because he loves me . . . every day is the best day.

ABOUT THE AUTHOR

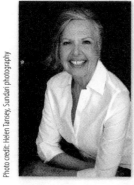

Photo credit: Helen Tansey, Sundari photography

Jocelyn Rasmussen is a singer, composer, and teacher. Her first book, *Meant to Be Heard*, maps the human voice and its potential for transformation. She has recorded two albums of original songs: *Just Love Away* and *Singing Is Praying Twice*. For over twenty years she taught singing and executive voice coaching in seminars and private sessions in New York City. She continues that work in Toronto and London, Ontario, where she lives with her partner, Doug Thompson.

Looking for your next great read?

We can help!

Visit www.shewritespress.com/next-read
or scan the QR code below for a list
of our recommended titles.

She Writes Press is an award-winning
independent publishing company founded to
serve women writers everywhere.